# DASH DIET

## Cookbook

## FOR BEGINNERS

A Complete Guide to Flavorful, Heart-Healthy Cooking. Including 14-day Meal Plan, Health Benefits and Full-Color Photos

BY

Gregory's Recipe Realm

# COPYRIGHT

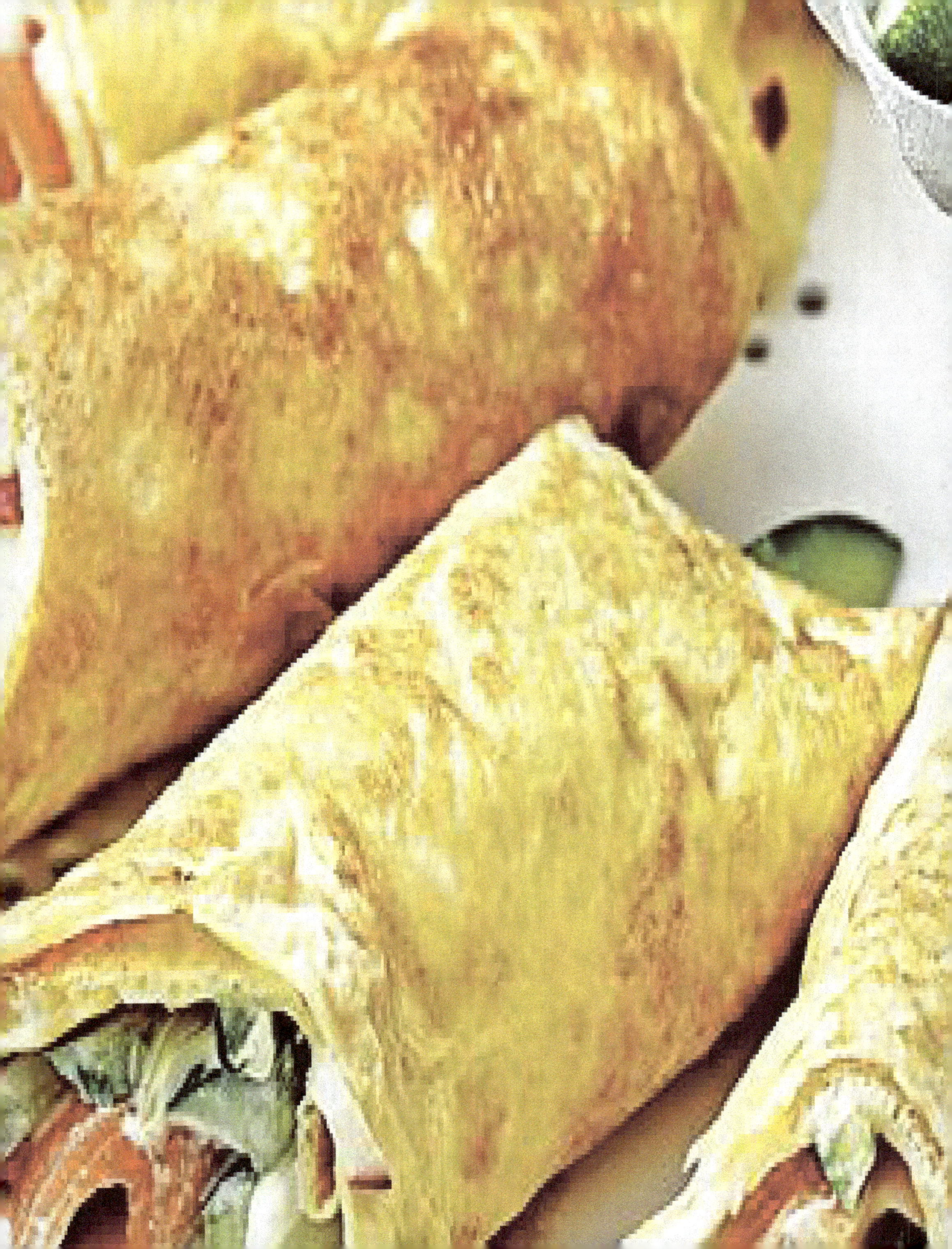

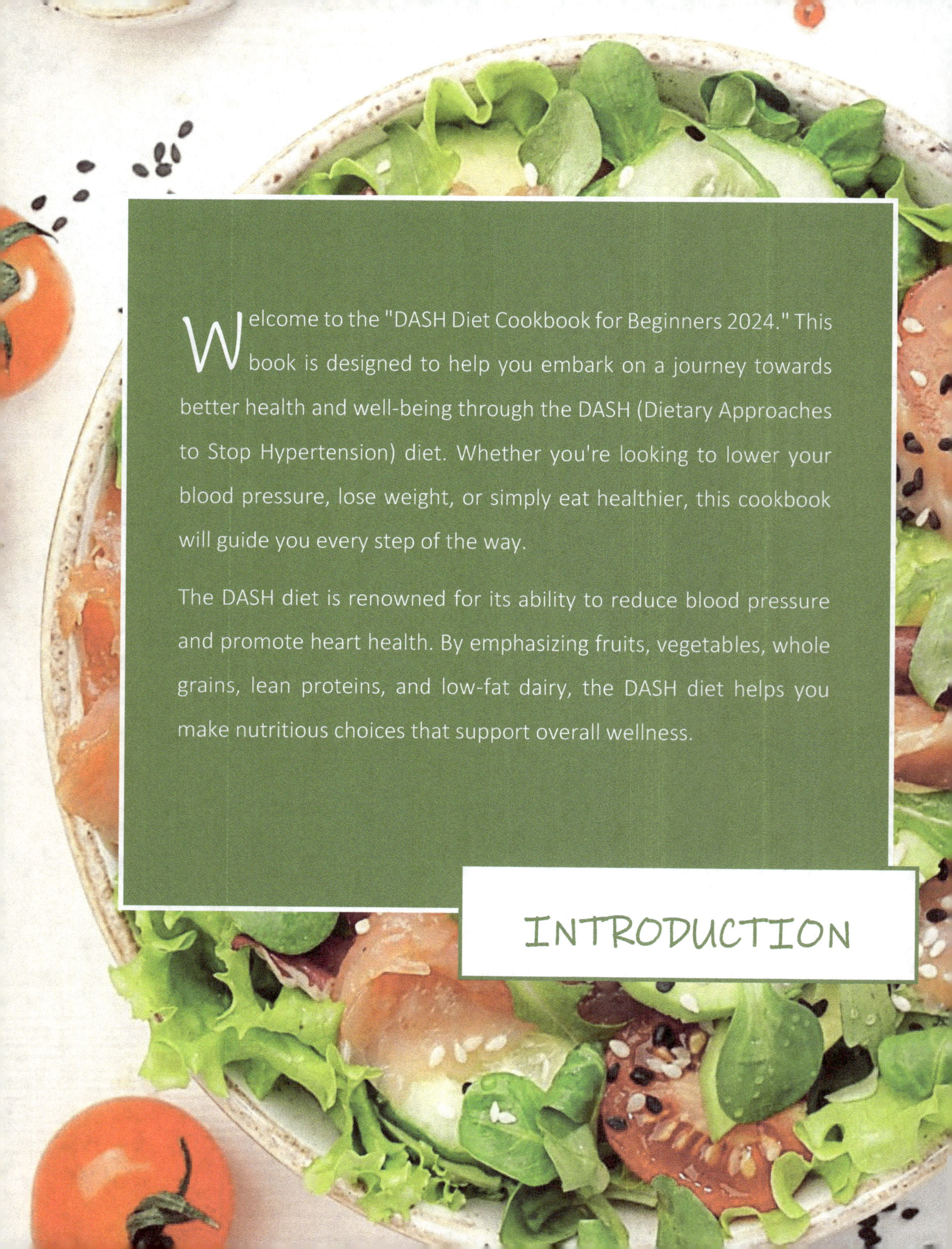

Welcome to the "DASH Diet Cookbook for Beginners 2024." This book is designed to help you embark on a journey towards better health and well-being through the DASH (Dietary Approaches to Stop Hypertension) diet. Whether you're looking to lower your blood pressure, lose weight, or simply eat healthier, this cookbook will guide you every step of the way.

The DASH diet is renowned for its ability to reduce blood pressure and promote heart health. By emphasizing fruits, vegetables, whole grains, lean proteins, and low-fat dairy, the DASH diet helps you make nutritious choices that support overall wellness.

# INTRODUCTION

# THE BENEFITS OF THE DASH DIET

## 1. LOWERING BLOOD PRESSURE

- **Hypertension Management:** The DASH diet was specifically designed to reduce blood pressure, a significant risk factor for heart disease and stroke. By emphasizing the consumption of fruits, vegetables, whole grains, lean proteins, and low-fat dairy while reducing sodium intake, the diet effectively lowers systolic and diastolic blood pressure.

- **Scientific Evidence:** Multiple studies have demonstrated the DASH diet's efficacy in reducing blood pressure. Research published in the New England Journal of Medicine showed that participants following the DASH diet experienced significant reductions in blood pressure compared to those on a typical American diet.

## 2. IMPROVING HEART HEALTH

- **Cholesterol Levels:** The DASH diet helps lower LDL (bad) cholesterol and triglycerides while raising HDL (good) cholesterol. This balanced approach to fat intake reduces the risk of atherosclerosis, heart attacks, and strokes.

- **Overall Cardiovascular Risk:** By promoting heart-healthy foods and reducing factors that contribute to cardiovascular disease, the DASH diet significantly lowers the overall risk of developing heart-related conditions.

## 3. PROMOTING WEIGHT LOSS AND MANAGEMENT

- Caloric Control: The DASH diet encourages portion control and the consumption of nutrient-dense foods, which can help individuals achieve and maintain a healthy weight. Unlike restrictive fad diets, the DASH diet promotes a balanced intake of calories, ensuring sustainable weight loss.

- Satiety and Cravings: High-fiber foods such as fruits, vegetables, and whole grains help increase feelings of fullness, reducing overeating and unhealthy snacking.

## 4. ENHANCING NUTRIENT INTAKE

- Nutrient-Dense Foods: The DASH diet emphasizes foods rich in essential nutrients like potassium, calcium, magnesium, and fiber. These nutrients are crucial for maintaining bodily functions, supporting bone health, and enhancing overall vitality.

- Antioxidants and Phytochemicals: A diet rich in fruits and vegetables provides a plethora of antioxidants and phytochemicals that protect against oxidative stress and inflammation, thereby reducing the risk of chronic diseases such as cancer and diabetes.

## 5. REDUCING THE RISK OF DIABETES

- **Blood Sugar Control:** The DASH diet's emphasis on whole grains, lean proteins, and healthy fats helps regulate blood sugar levels. This balanced approach can prevent insulin resistance, a precursor to type 2 diabetes.

- **Prevention and Management:** For individuals with prediabetes or diabetes, the DASH diet offers a practical and effective way to manage blood sugar levels and prevent complications associated with the disease.

## 6. SUPPORTING KIDNEY HEALTH

- **Reduced Sodium Intake:** High sodium intake is a major contributor to kidney disease. The DASH diet's low sodium guidelines help prevent kidney damage and support overall renal health.

- **Improved Kidney Function:** The emphasis on potassium-rich foods aids in balancing sodium levels, thereby reducing strain on the kidneys and improving their function.

## 7. ENHANCING MENTAL HEALTH

- Mood and Cognitive Function: Nutrient-rich foods, such as leafy greens, fatty fish, and nuts, provide essential fatty acids and vitamins that support brain health. Improved nutrition can enhance mood, cognitive function, and reduce the risk of mental health disorders.

- Stress Reduction: By regulating blood pressure and improving overall health, the DASH diet can also contribute to reduced stress levels, further promoting mental well-being.

# UNDERSTANDING DASH DIET PRINCIPLES

## 1. EMPHASIS ON FRUITS AND VEGETABLES

Incorporating plenty of fruits and vegetables is central to the DASH diet. These foods are rich in essential nutrients like potassium, magnesium, and fiber, which are crucial for maintaining healthy blood pressure and overall health.

## 2. INCLUSION OF WHOLE GRAINS

Whole grains such as brown rice, quinoa, oats, and whole wheat are prioritized over refined grains. They provide sustained energy and essential nutrients, including fiber, which supports digestive health and helps regulate blood sugar levels.

### 3. LEAN PROTEIN SOURCES

The DASH diet encourages lean protein sources, including poultry, fish, beans, and nuts, while limiting red and processed meats. Lean proteins are important for muscle maintenance and overall body function without contributing excessive saturated fats.

### 4. LOW-FAT AND NON-FAT DAIRY

Low-fat and non-fat dairy products like milk, yogurt, and cheese are recommended. These are good sources of calcium and vitamin D, which are vital for bone health and can aid in blood pressure regulation.

### 5. REDUCED SODIUM INTAKE

One of the key strategies of the DASH diet is to reduce sodium intake to less than 2,300 milligrams per day, and ideally to 1,500 milligrams for greater blood pressure reduction. This involves choosing fresh, unprocessed foods and being mindful of sodium content in packaged foods.

# ESSENTIAL INGREDIENTS FOR YOUR KITCHEN

## FRUITS AND VEGETABLES

- Fresh: Apples, berries, oranges, leafy greens, tomatoes, bell peppers, carrots
- Frozen: Mixed vegetables, berries, peas
- Whole Grains
- Brown rice
- Quinoa
- Oats
- Whole wheat bread and pasta
- Lean Proteins
- Skinless chicken breasts
- Fish (salmon, tuna)
- Beans (black beans, chickpeas)
- Lentils
- Tofu
- Low-Fat and Non-Fat Dairy
- Skim milk or 1% milk
- Greek yogurt
- Low-fat cheese
- Healthy Fats
- Olive oil
- Avocados
- Nuts and seeds (almonds, walnuts, chia seeds)
- Seasonings and Spices
- Garlic
- Herbs (basil, cilantro, parsley)

- Spices (turmeric, paprika, cumin)
- Lemon and lime juice
- Healthy Snacks
- Fresh fruit
- Vegetable sticks with hummus
- Nuts and seeds

- Pantry Staples
- Canned tomatoes (no added salt)
- Low-sodium broth
- Whole grain cereals
- Natural nut butters

*Having these ingredients readily available will help you prepare nutritious, DASH-friendly meals with ease, ensuring you stay on track with your dietary goals.*

## ESSENTIAL TOOLS

- **Sharp Knives:** For efficient and safe food preparation.
- **Cutting Boards:** Separate boards for fruits/vegetables and meats to avoid cross-contamination.
- **Measuring Cups and Spoons:** For accurate portion control.

- **Blender/Food Processor:** Useful for smoothies, soups, and sauces.
- **Non-Stick Pans:** To reduce the need for added fats.
- **Slow Cooker/Instant Pot:** For convenient, healthy meal preparation.
- **Storage Containers:** For meal prep and portioning out snacks and meals.

## TIPS FOR SUCCESS

- **Meal Planning:** Plan your meals and snacks for the week to ensure balanced nutrition and avoid last-minute unhealthy choices.
- **Grocery Shopping List:** Make a list before shopping to stay focused and avoid buying unhealthy foods.

- **Batch Cooking:** Prepare large batches of meals to save time and ensure you have healthy options readily available.
- **Stay Hydrated:** Drink plenty of water throughout the day to support overall health.

- **Read Labels:** Check nutrition labels for sodium, sugar, and unhealthy fats, and choose the healthiest options.
- **Mindful Eating:** Eat slowly and pay attention to hunger and fullness cues to avoid overeating.
- **Physical Activity:** Incorporate regular physical activity to complement your healthy eating habits and improve overall well-being.
- **Seek Support:** Join a support group or find a diet buddy to stay motivated and share tips and experiences.

*By equipping your kitchen with the right tools and following these tips, you'll create a supportive environment that makes sticking to the DASH diet both manageable and enjoyable.*

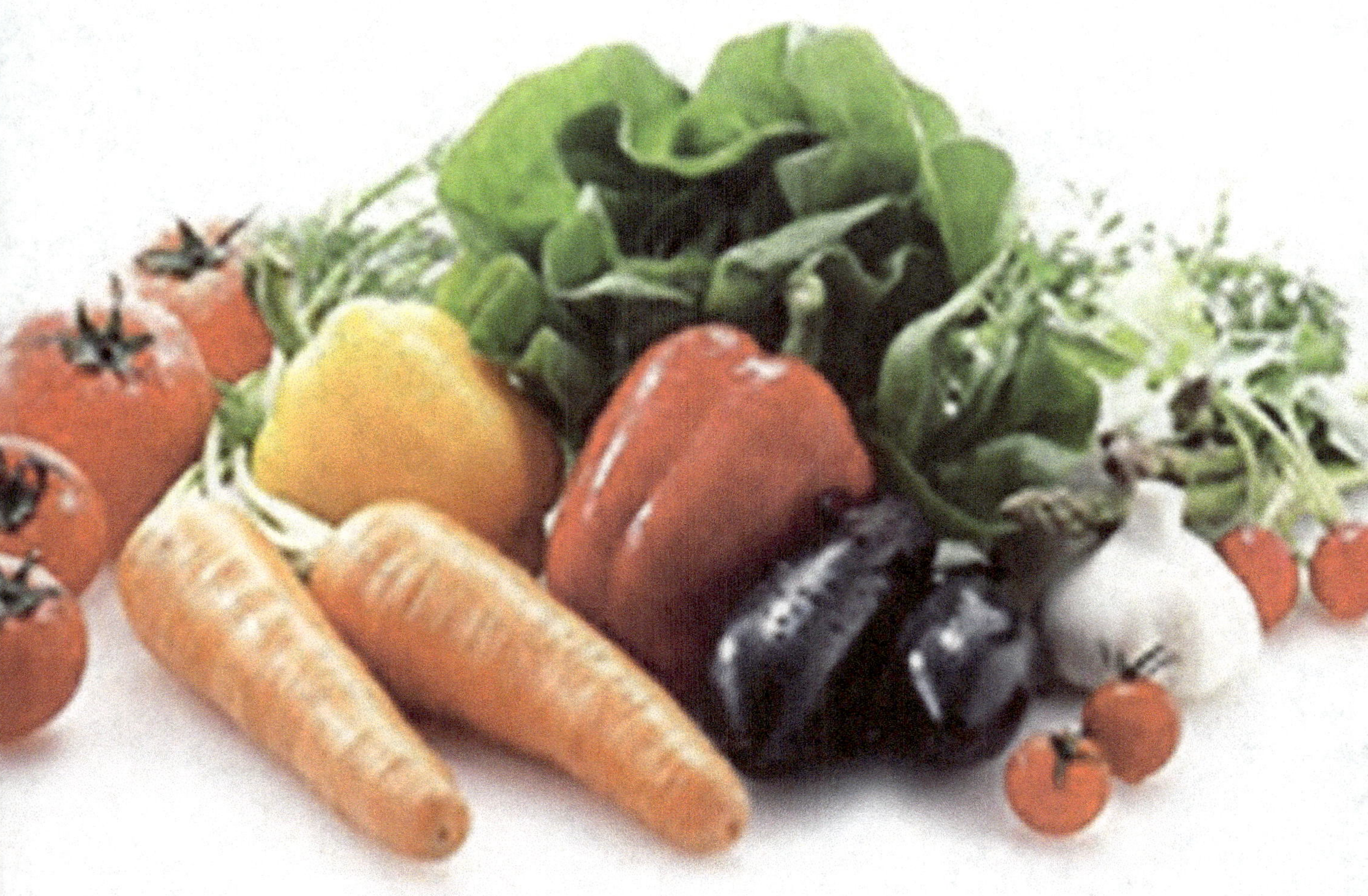

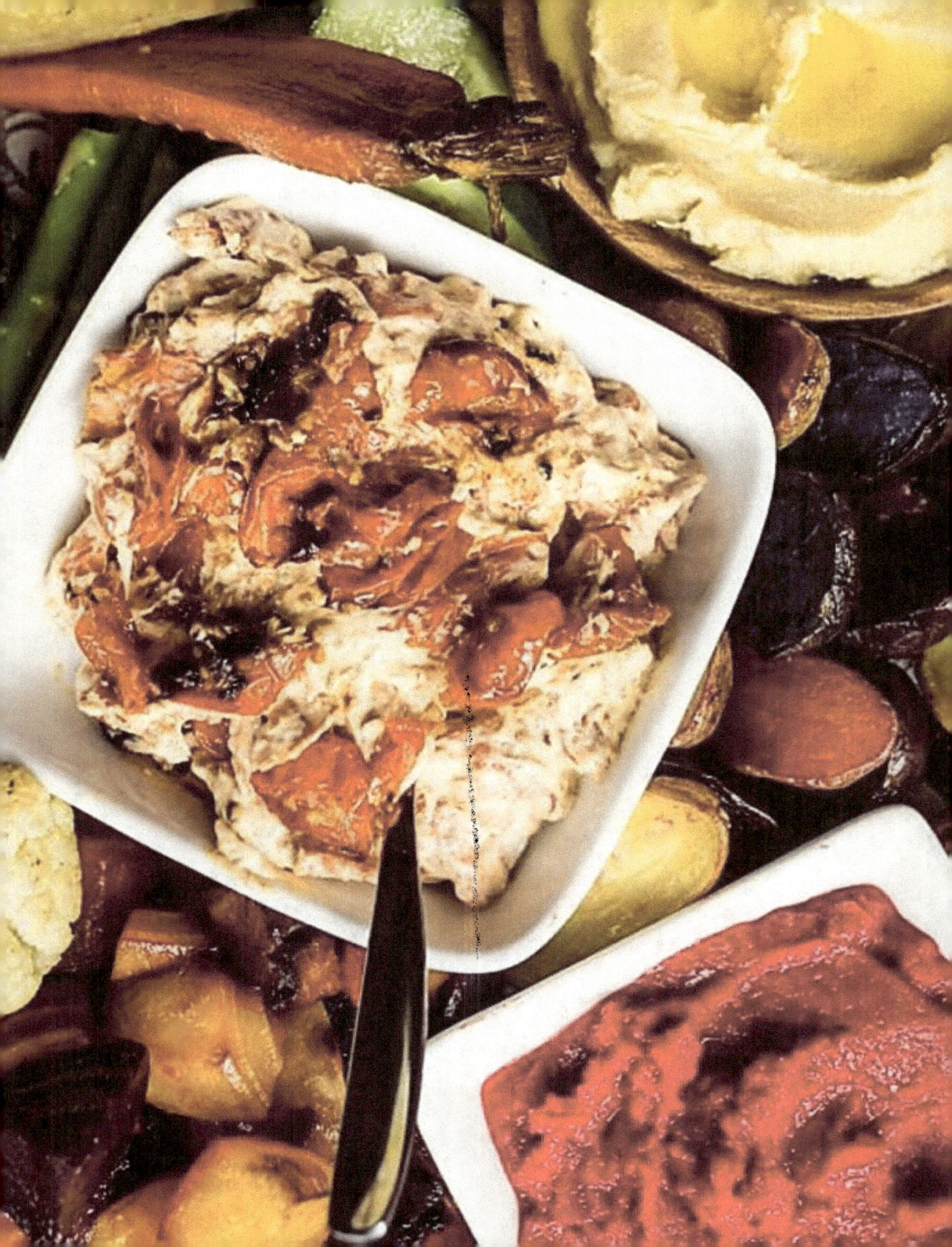

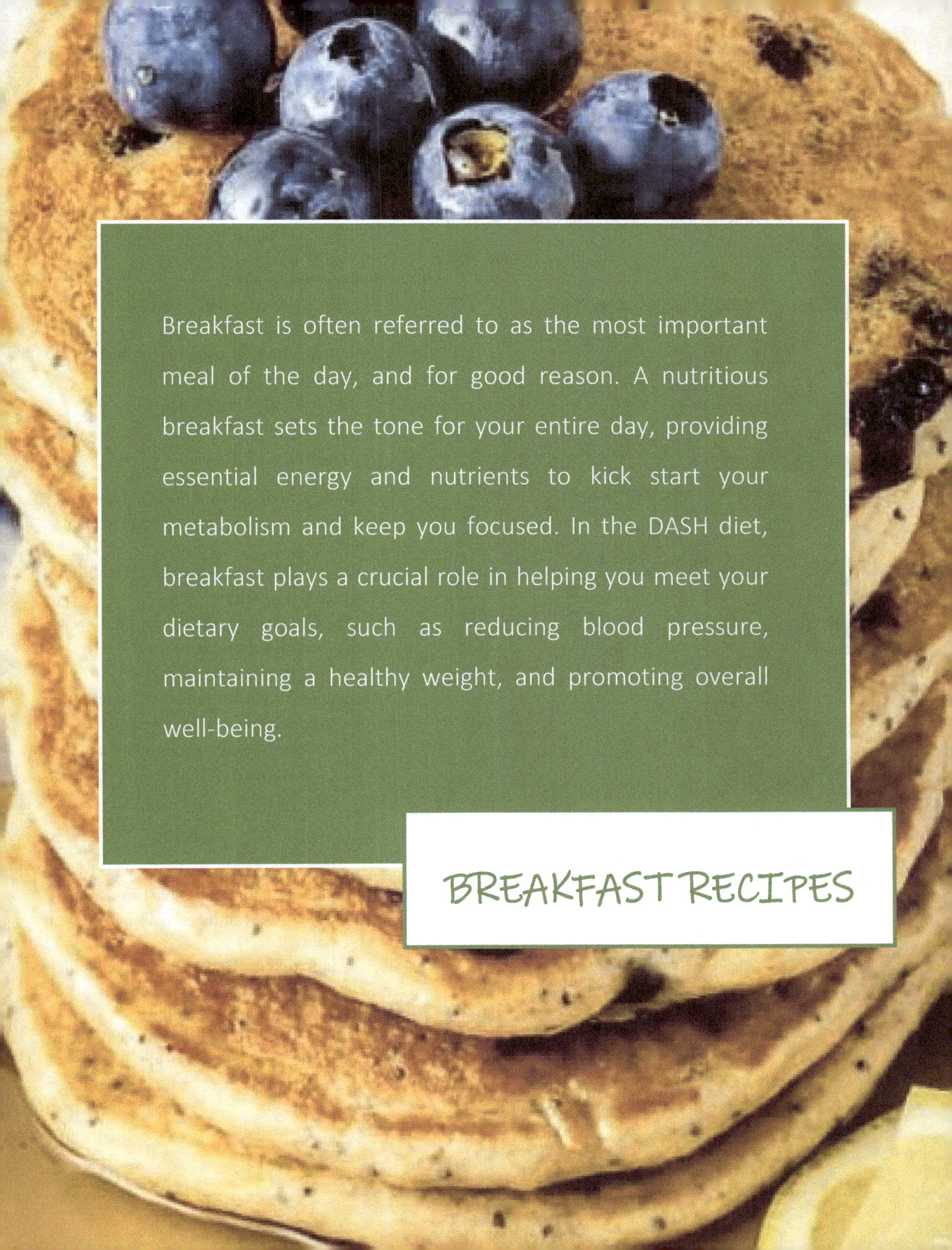

Breakfast is often referred to as the most important meal of the day, and for good reason. A nutritious breakfast sets the tone for your entire day, providing essential energy and nutrients to kick start your metabolism and keep you focused. In the DASH diet, breakfast plays a crucial role in helping you meet your dietary goals, such as reducing blood pressure, maintaining a healthy weight, and promoting overall well-being.

BREAKFAST RECIPES

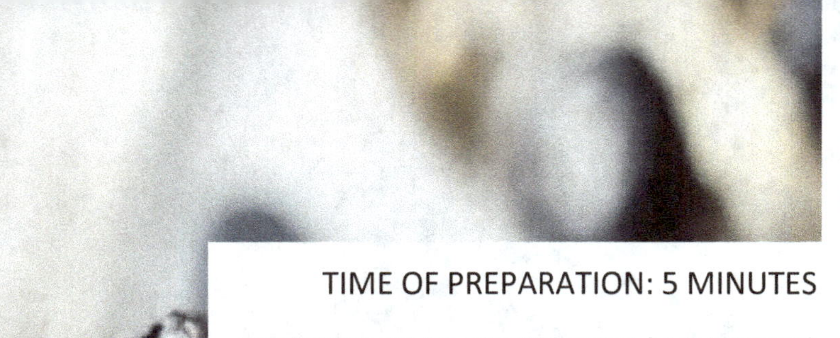

TIME OF PREPARATION: 5 MINUTES

COOKING TIME: OVERNIGHT (6-8 HOURS)

SERVING UNIT: 1 SERVING

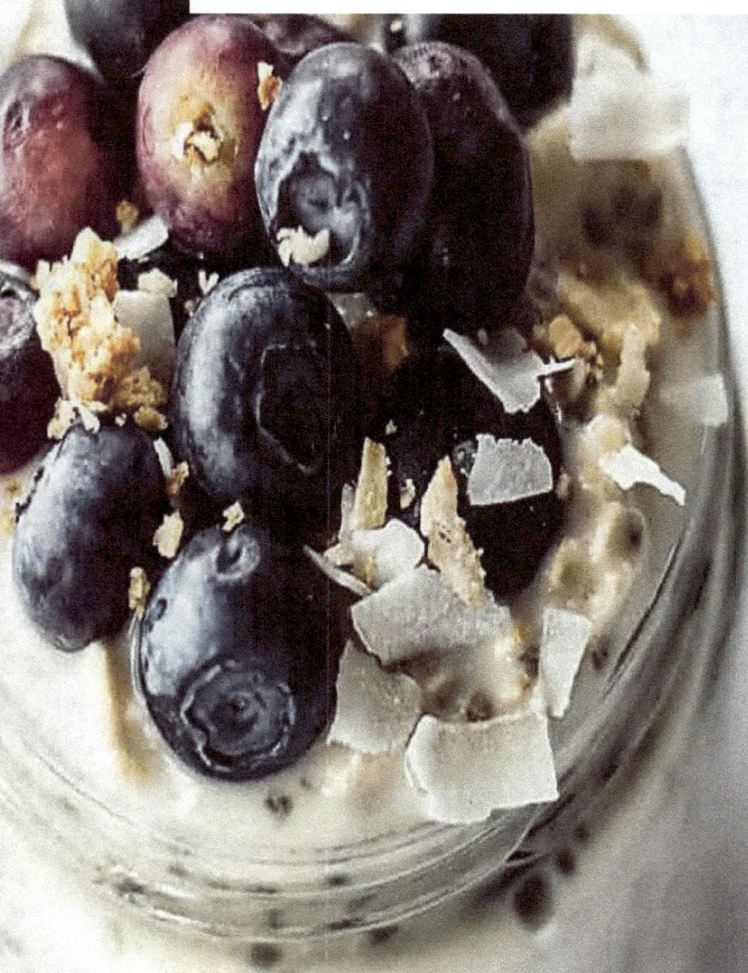

# BERRY OVERNIGHT OATS

- 1/2 cup rolled oats
- 1/2 cup unsweetened almond milk (or any milk of choice)
- 1/4 cup Greek yogurt
- 1/2 cup mixed berries (strawberries, blueberries, raspberries)
- 1 tablespoon honey or maple syrup (optional)
- 1 tablespoon chia seeds (optional)
- A pinch of cinnamon (optional)

## PROCEDURES

1. In a mason jar or bowl, combine rolled oats, almond milk, Greek yogurt, and honey/maple syrup if using.
2. Stir in chia seeds and cinnamon, if desired, for added texture and flavor.
3. Gently fold in mixed berries, ensuring they are evenly distributed throughout the mixture.
4. Cover the jar or bowl and refrigerate overnight, or for at least 6-8 hours, to allow the oats to soften and the flavors to meld.
5. In the morning, give the oats a good stir and enjoy cold or warmed up in the microwave for a cozy breakfast treat.

## HEALTH BENEFITS

1. High in fiber: Supports digestive health and promotes feelings of fullness, aiding in weight management.
2. Rich in antioxidants: Berries are packed with antioxidants that help protect cells from damage and reduce inflammation.
3. Balanced nutrition: Provides a good balance of carbohydrates, protein, and healthy fats to sustain energy levels throughout the morning.

## NUTRITIONAL VALUES

CALORIES: 300 KCAL | PROTEIN: 12G | FAT: 6G | CARBOHYDRATES: 50G | FIBER: 8G | SUGAR: 12G

# SPINACH AND FETA OMELET

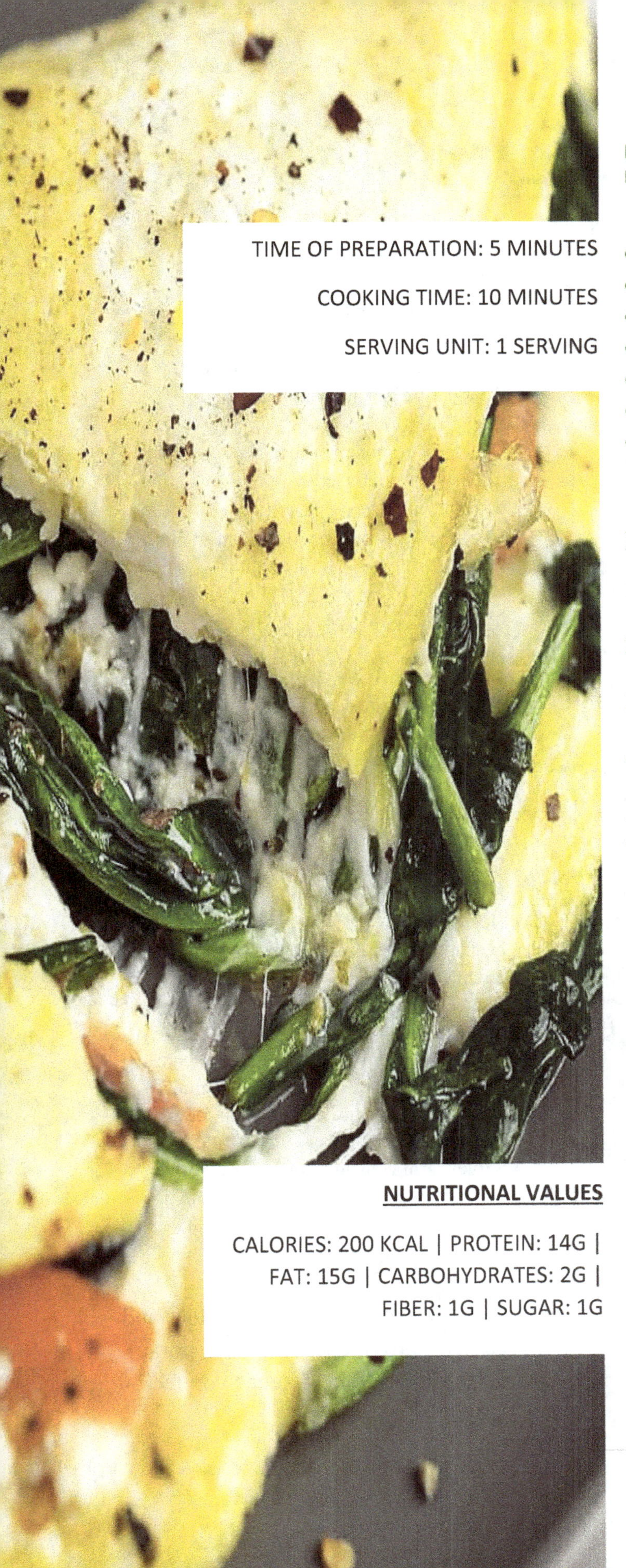

TIME OF PREPARATION: 5 MINUTES

COOKING TIME: 10 MINUTES

SERVING UNIT: 1 SERVING

- 2 large eggs
- 1/4 cup fresh spinach, chopped
- 2 tablespoons feta cheese, crumbled
- 1 tablespoon milk (optional)
- 1 tablespoon olive oil or cooking spray
- Salt and pepper, to taste
- Fresh herbs (such as parsley or dill), optional for garnish

## PROCEDURES

1. In a small bowl, whisk together the eggs, milk (if using), salt, and pepper until well combined.
2. Heat olive oil in a non-stick skillet over medium heat.
3. Add the chopped spinach to the skillet and sauté for 1-2 minutes until wilted.
4. Pour the egg mixture over the spinach, tilting the pan to spread it evenly.
5. Sprinkle the feta cheese evenly over the eggs.
6. Cook the omelet without stirring until the edges start to set, about 2-3 minutes.
7. Carefully fold the omelet in half and continue cooking for another 2-3 minutes until fully set.
8. Slide the omelet onto a plate, garnish with fresh herbs if desired, and serve immediately.

## HEALTH BENEFITS

1. High in protein: Eggs are an excellent source of high-quality protein, essential for muscle repair and maintenance.
2. Rich in vitamins and minerals: Spinach provides a wealth of vitamins A, C, and K, as well as iron and calcium, which are vital for overall health.
3. Good source of healthy fats: Feta cheese and olive oil contribute to healthy fats that support heart health and provide sustained energy.

### NUTRITIONAL VALUES

CALORIES: 200 KCAL | PROTEIN: 14G | FAT: 15G | CARBOHYDRATES: 2G | FIBER: 1G | SUGAR: 1G

# BANANA NUT PANCAKES

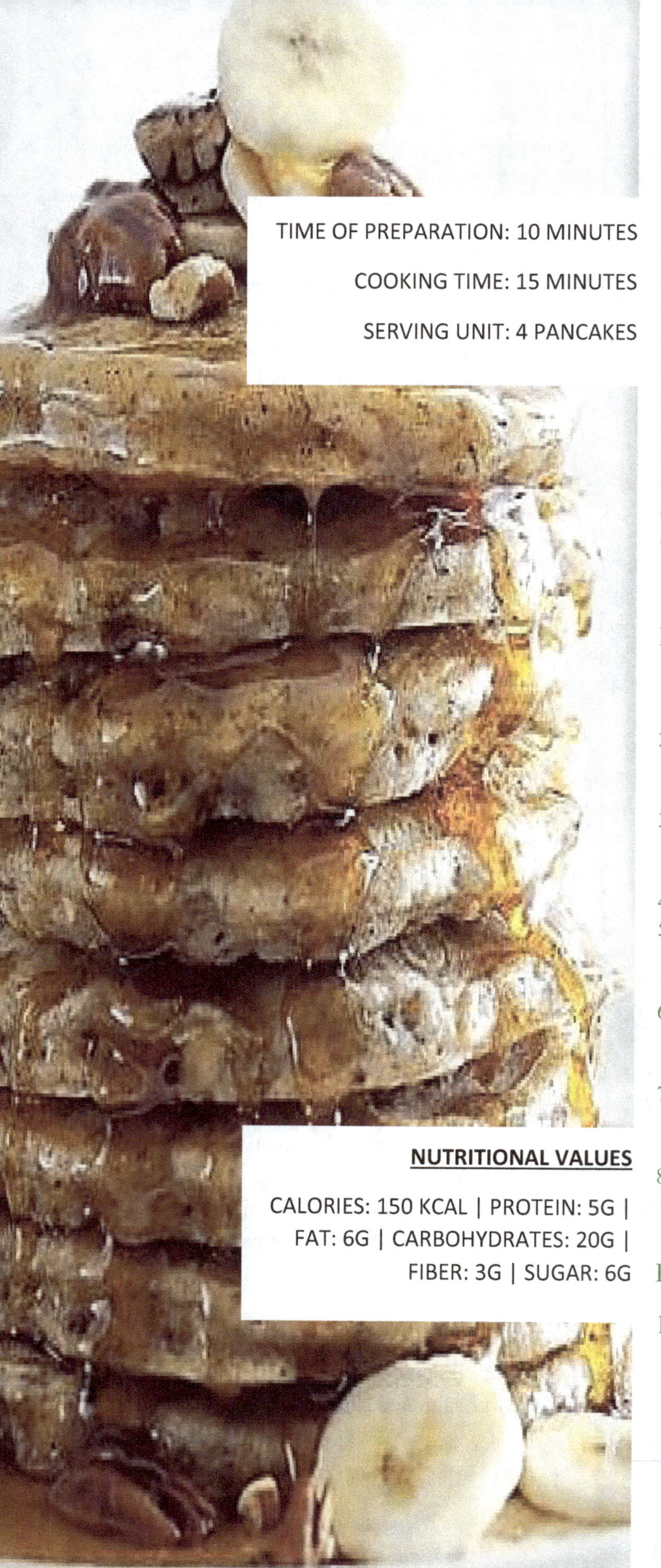

TIME OF PREPARATION: 10 MINUTES

COOKING TIME: 15 MINUTES

SERVING UNIT: 4 PANCAKES

- 1 cup whole wheat flour
- 1 tablespoon baking powder
- 1/2 teaspoon cinnamon
- 1/4 teaspoon salt
- 1 cup almond milk (or any milk of choice)
- 1 large ripe banana, mashed
- 1 egg
- 1 tablespoon honey or maple syrup
- 1 teaspoon vanilla extract
- 1/4 cup chopped walnuts
- Cooking spray or a small amount of butter for the pan

## PROCEDURES

1. In a large bowl, whisk together the flour, baking powder, cinnamon, and salt.
2. In a separate bowl, combine the almond milk, mashed banana, egg, honey or maple syrup, and vanilla extract. Mix well.
3. Pour the wet ingredients into the dry ingredients and stir until just combined. Do not overmix; the batter should be slightly lumpy.
4. Fold in the chopped walnuts.
5. Heat a non-stick skillet or griddle over medium heat and lightly grease with cooking spray or butter.
6. Pour 1/4 cup of batter onto the skillet for each pancake. Cook until bubbles form on the surface and the edges look set, about 2-3 minutes.
7. Flip the pancakes and cook for an additional 2-3 minutes, or until golden brown and cooked through.
8. Serve warm with additional banana slices, walnuts, and a drizzle of honey or maple syrup, if desired.

**NUTRITIONAL VALUES**

CALORIES: 150 KCAL | PROTEIN: 5G | FAT: 6G | CARBOHYDRATES: 20G | FIBER: 3G | SUGAR: 6G

## HEALTH BENEFITS

1. High in fiber: Whole wheat flour and bananas provide fiber that supports digestive health and keeps you feeling full longer.

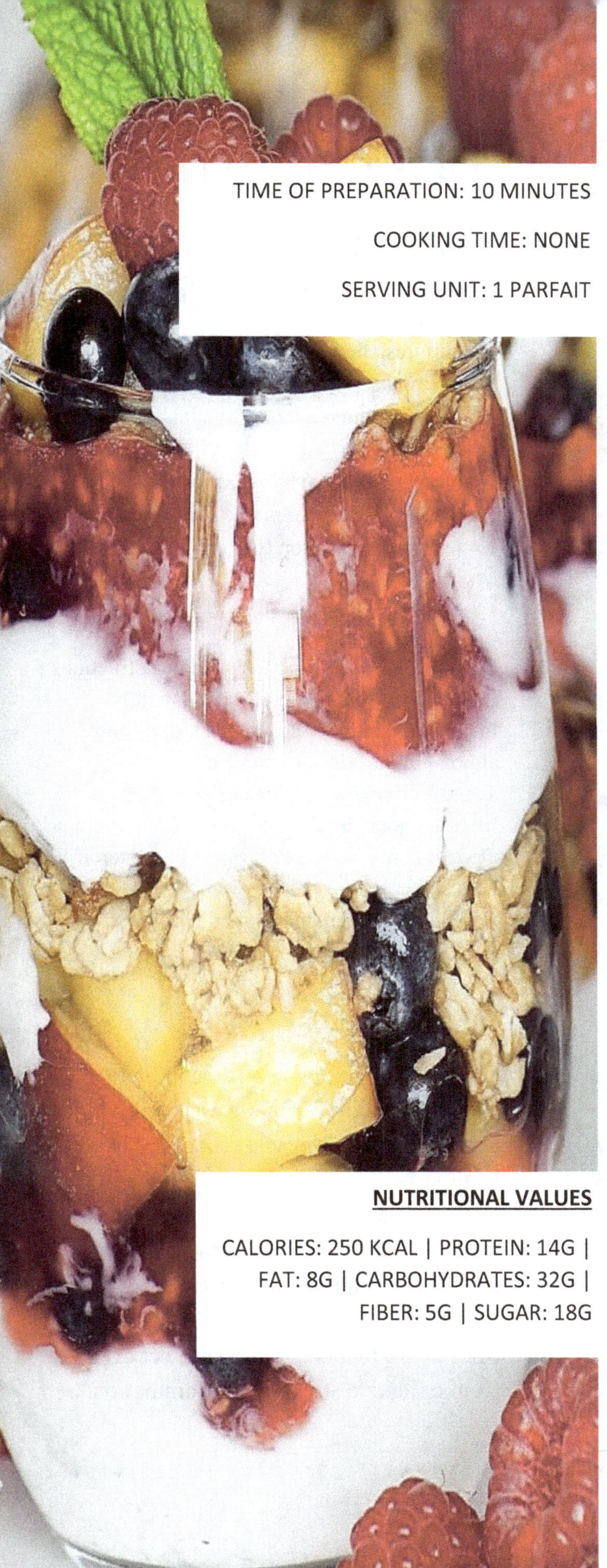



# GREEK YOGURT PARFAIT WITH FRESH FRUITS

- 1 cup Greek yogurt (plain or vanilla)
- 1/2 cup fresh mixed berries (strawberries, blueberries, raspberries)
- 1/4 cup granola
- 1 tablespoon honey or maple syrup (optional)
- 1 tablespoon chia seeds or flaxseeds (optional)
- Fresh mint leaves for garnish (optional)

## PROCEDURES

2. Spoon half of the Greek yogurt into a serving glass or bowl.
3. Layer half of the mixed berries on top of the yogurt.
4. Add a layer of granola over the berries.
5. Repeat the layers with the remaining yogurt and berries.
6. Drizzle honey or maple syrup over the top, if desired.
7. Sprinkle chia seeds or flaxseeds on top for added nutrition.
8. Garnish with fresh mint leaves if using.
9. Serve immediately and enjoy.

## HEALTH BENEFITS

1. High in protein: Greek yogurt provides a substantial amount of protein, which helps build and repair tissues and keeps you feeling full longer.
2. Rich in probiotics: Greek yogurt contains probiotics that support a healthy gut microbiome and improve digestion.

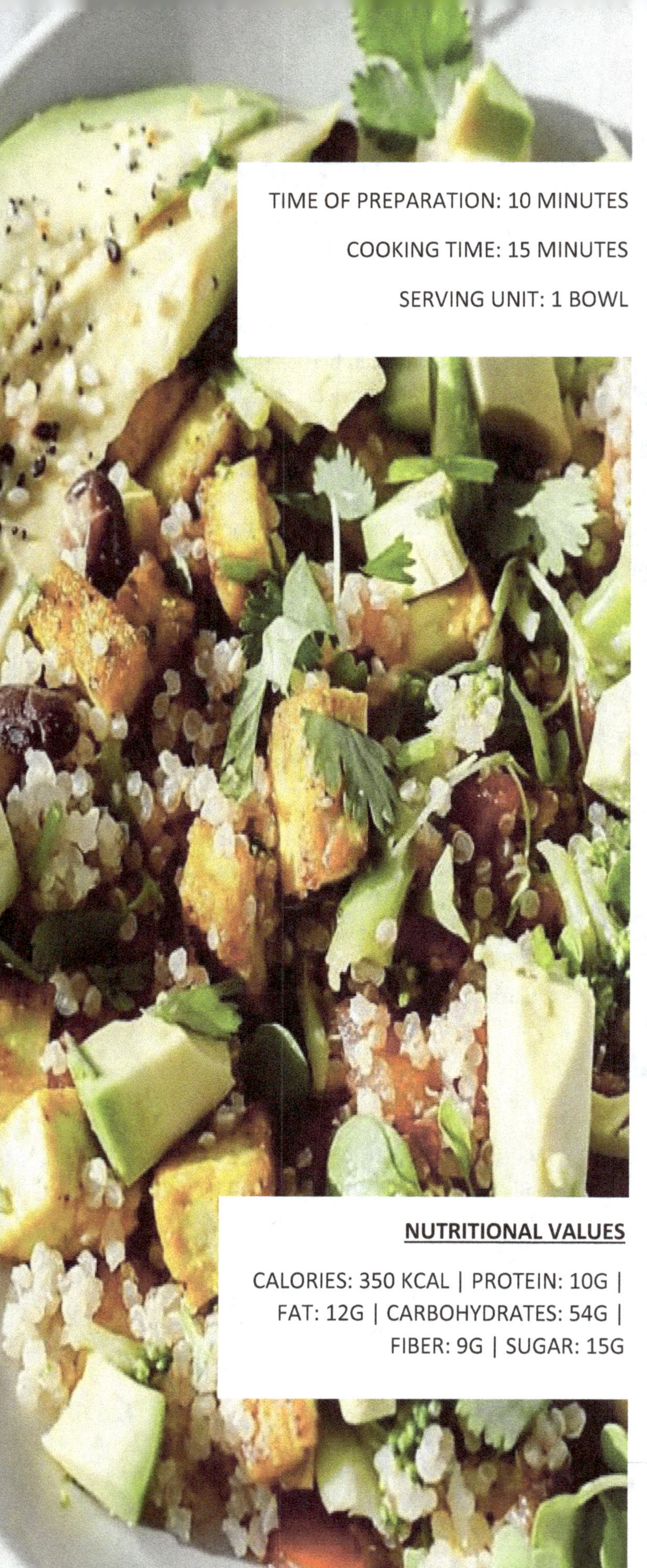

TIME OF PREPARATION: 10 MINUTES

COOKING TIME: 15 MINUTES

SERVING UNIT: 1 BOWL

**NUTRITIONAL VALUES**

CALORIES: 350 KCAL | PROTEIN: 10G |
FAT: 12G | CARBOHYDRATES: 54G |
FIBER: 9G | SUGAR: 15G

# QUINOA BREAKFAST BOWL

- 1/2 cup cooked quinoa
- 1/4 cup almond milk (or any milk of choice)
- 1/2 banana, sliced
- 1/4 cup fresh berries (blueberries, strawberries, or raspberries)
- 1 tablespoon nuts (almonds, walnuts, or pecans), chopped
- 1 tablespoon seeds (chia seeds or flaxseeds)
- 1 tablespoon honey or maple syrup (optional)
- 1/4 teaspoon cinnamon (optional)

## PROCEDURES

1. Cook quinoa according to package instructions if not already cooked. Let it cool slightly.
2. In a bowl, combine the cooked quinoa and almond milk. Stir to mix evenly.
3. Top the quinoa with banana slices, fresh berries, chopped nuts, and seeds.
4. Drizzle honey or maple syrup over the top if desired.
5. Sprinkle with cinnamon for added flavor.
6. Serve immediately and enjoy.

## HEALTH BENEFITS

1. High in protein: Quinoa is a complete protein, providing all nine essential amino acids, crucial for muscle repair and overall health.
2. Rich in fiber: This bowl is loaded with fiber from quinoa, fruits, and seeds, aiding in digestion and promoting satiety.
3. Packed with antioxidants: Fresh berries offer antioxidants that help protect cells from oxidative stress and inflammation.

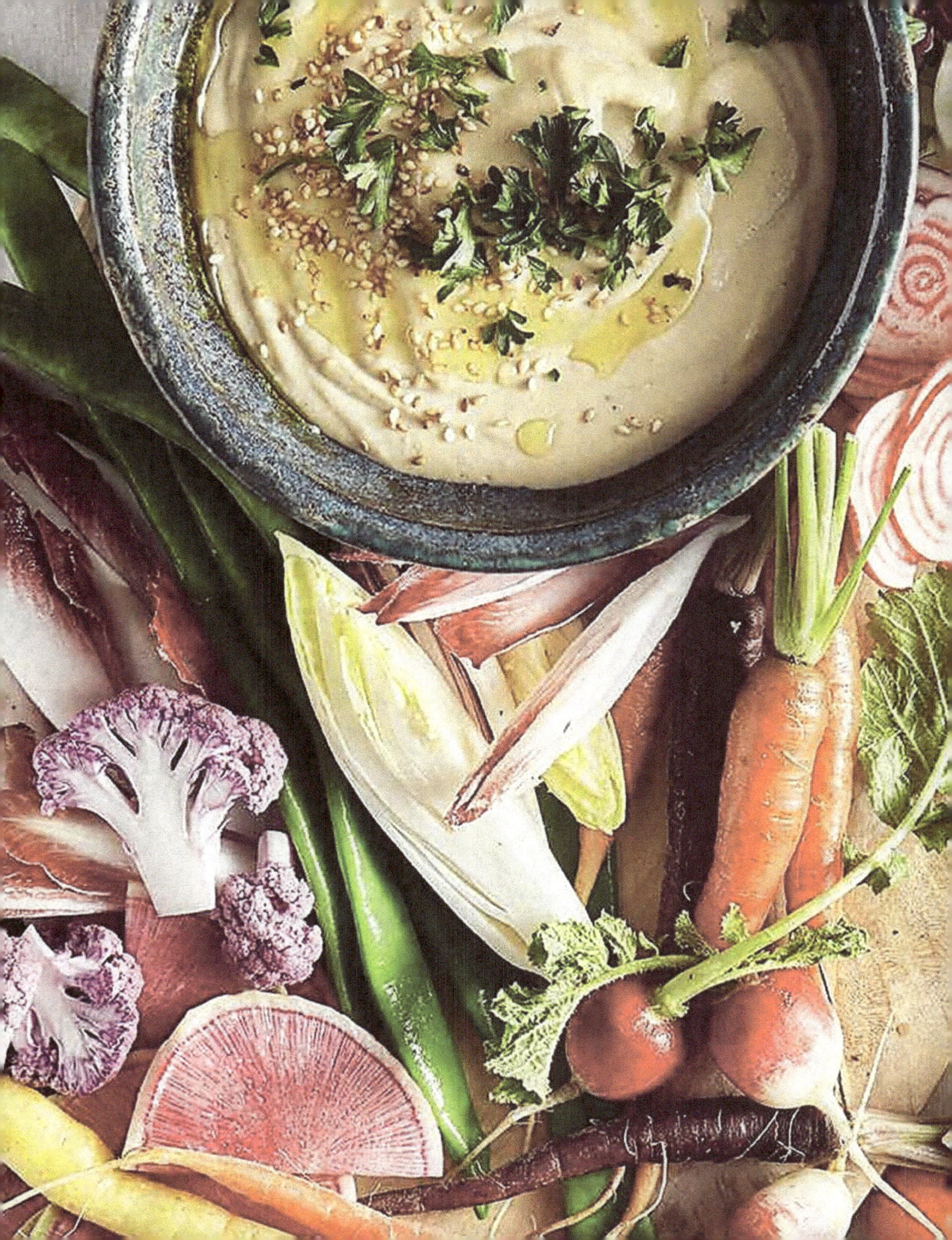

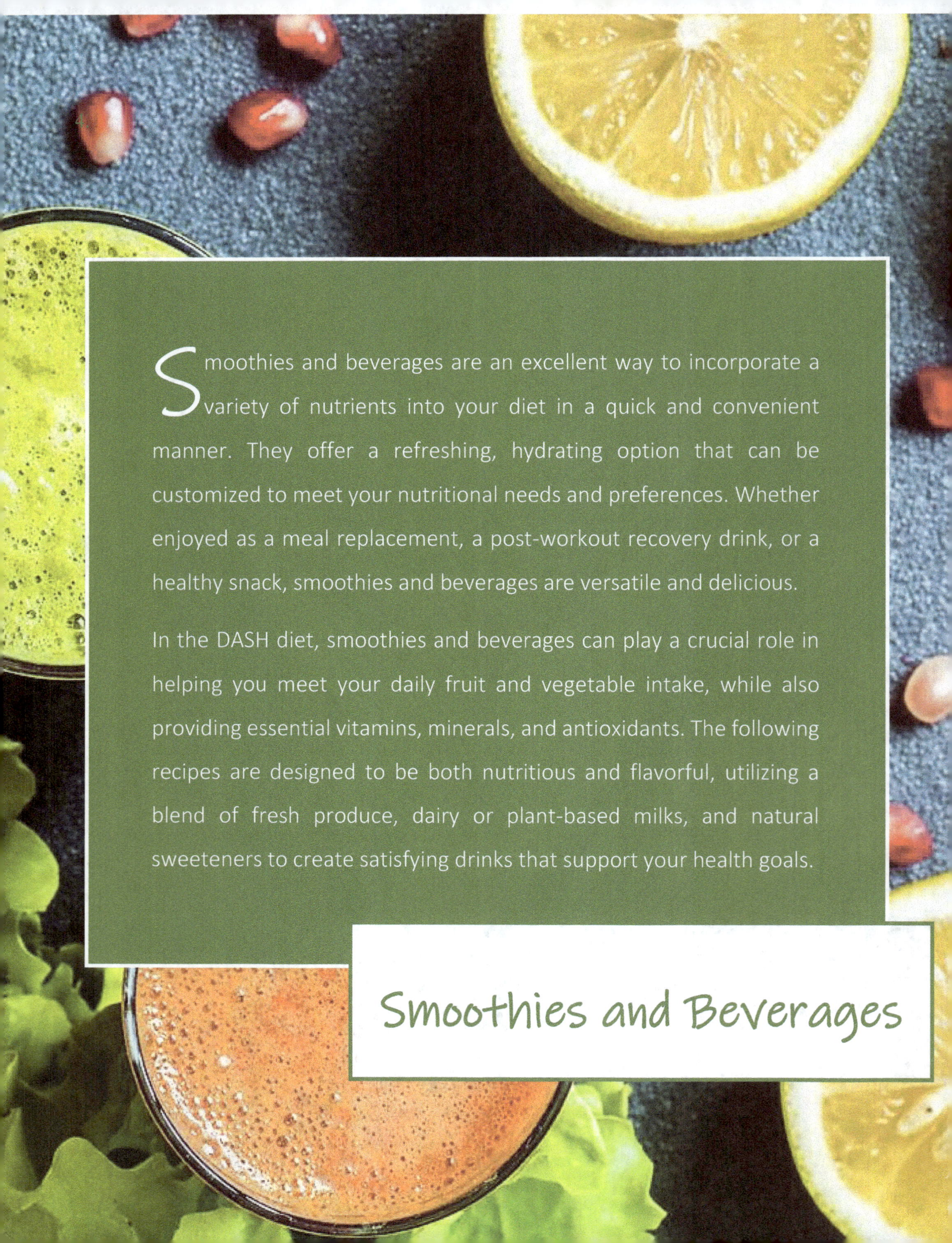

Smoothies and beverages are an excellent way to incorporate a variety of nutrients into your diet in a quick and convenient manner. They offer a refreshing, hydrating option that can be customized to meet your nutritional needs and preferences. Whether enjoyed as a meal replacement, a post-workout recovery drink, or a healthy snack, smoothies and beverages are versatile and delicious.

In the DASH diet, smoothies and beverages can play a crucial role in helping you meet your daily fruit and vegetable intake, while also providing essential vitamins, minerals, and antioxidants. The following recipes are designed to be both nutritious and flavorful, utilizing a blend of fresh produce, dairy or plant-based milks, and natural sweeteners to create satisfying drinks that support your health goals.

# Smoothies and Beverages

# BERRY BLAST SMOOTHIE

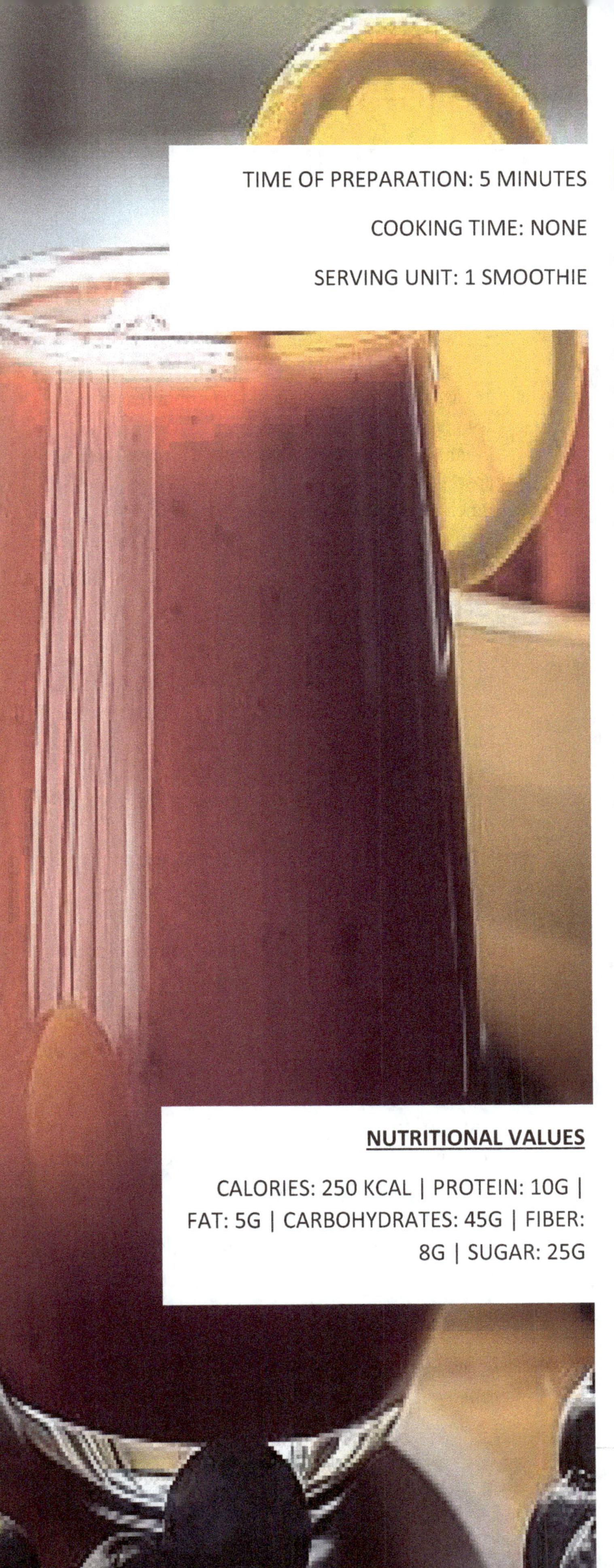

TIME OF PREPARATION: 5 MINUTES

COOKING TIME: NONE

SERVING UNIT: 1 SMOOTHIE

- 1 cup mixed berries (strawberries, blueberries, raspberries, blackberries)
- 1/2 banana
- 1/2 cup Greek yogurt
- 1/2 cup almond milk (or any milk of choice)
- 1 tablespoon honey or maple syrup (optional)
- 1 tablespoon chia seeds or flaxseeds (optional)
- 1/2 teaspoon vanilla extract (optional)
- Ice cubes (optional, for a thicker smoothie)

## PROCEDURES

1. Place mixed berries, banana, Greek yogurt, and almond milk into a blender.
2. Add honey or maple syrup, chia seeds or flaxseeds, and vanilla extract if using.
3. Blend on high until smooth and creamy.
4. If a thicker consistency is desired, add a few ice cubes and blend again until smooth.
5. Pour into a glass and serve immediately.

## HEALTH BENEFITS

1. High in antioxidants: Berries are rich in antioxidants, which protect cells from oxidative stress and inflammation.
2. Good source of fiber: This smoothie is packed with fiber from fruits and seeds, supporting digestive health and promoting fullness.
3. Protein boost: Greek yogurt provides protein, essential for muscle repair and maintenance.

### NUTRITIONAL VALUES

CALORIES: 250 KCAL | PROTEIN: 10G | FAT: 5G | CARBOHYDRATES: 45G | FIBER: 8G | SUGAR: 25G

# GOLDEN TURMERIC LATTE

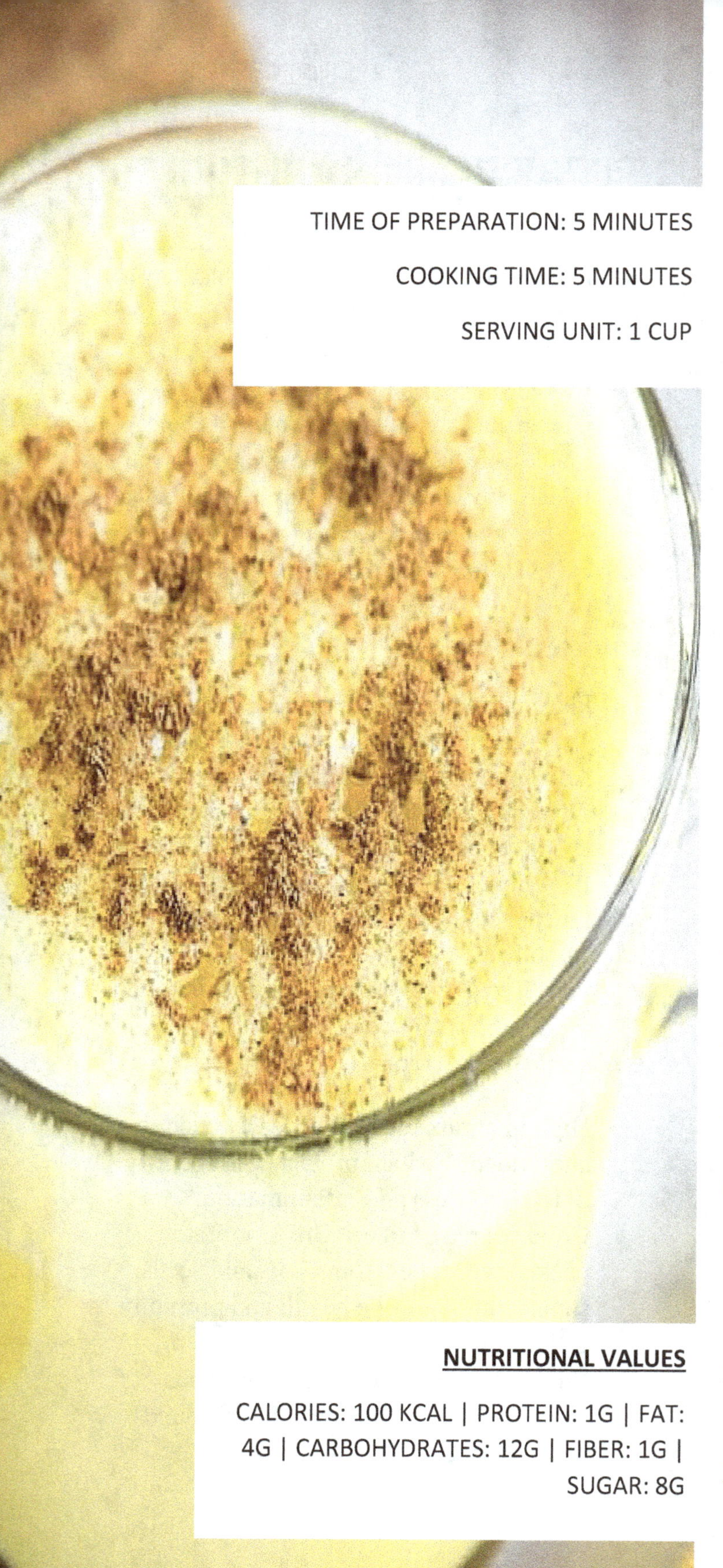

TIME OF PREPARATION: 5 MINUTES

COOKING TIME: 5 MINUTES

SERVING UNIT: 1 CUP

- 1 cup unsweetened almond milk (or any milk of choice)
- 1 teaspoon ground turmeric
- 1/2 teaspoon ground cinnamon
- 1/4 teaspoon ground ginger
- 1 teaspoon honey or maple syrup (optional)
- 1/4 teaspoon vanilla extract (optional)
- Pinch of black pepper (enhances turmeric absorption)
- Pinch of ground nutmeg (optional)
- 1 teaspoon coconut oil (optional, for added creaminess)

## PROCEDURES

1. In a small saucepan, combine almond milk, turmeric, cinnamon, ginger, black pepper, and nutmeg (if using).
2. Heat over medium heat, stirring constantly, until the mixture is hot but not boiling, about 3-5 minutes.
3. Remove from heat and stir in honey or maple syrup, vanilla extract, and coconut oil (if using).
4. Whisk vigorously or use a milk frother to create a frothy consistency.
5. Pour into a mug and serve immediately.

## HEALTH BENEFITS

1. Anti-inflammatory properties: Turmeric contains curcumin, a powerful anti-inflammatory compound that can help reduce inflammation and joint pain.
2. Antioxidant-rich: The spices in this latte are rich in antioxidants, which protect cells from damage and support overall health.
3. Digestive support: Ginger and turmeric are known to aid digestion and soothe the digestive tract.

## NUTRITIONAL VALUES

CALORIES: 100 KCAL | PROTEIN: 1G | FAT: 4G | CARBOHYDRATES: 12G | FIBER: 1G | SUGAR: 8G

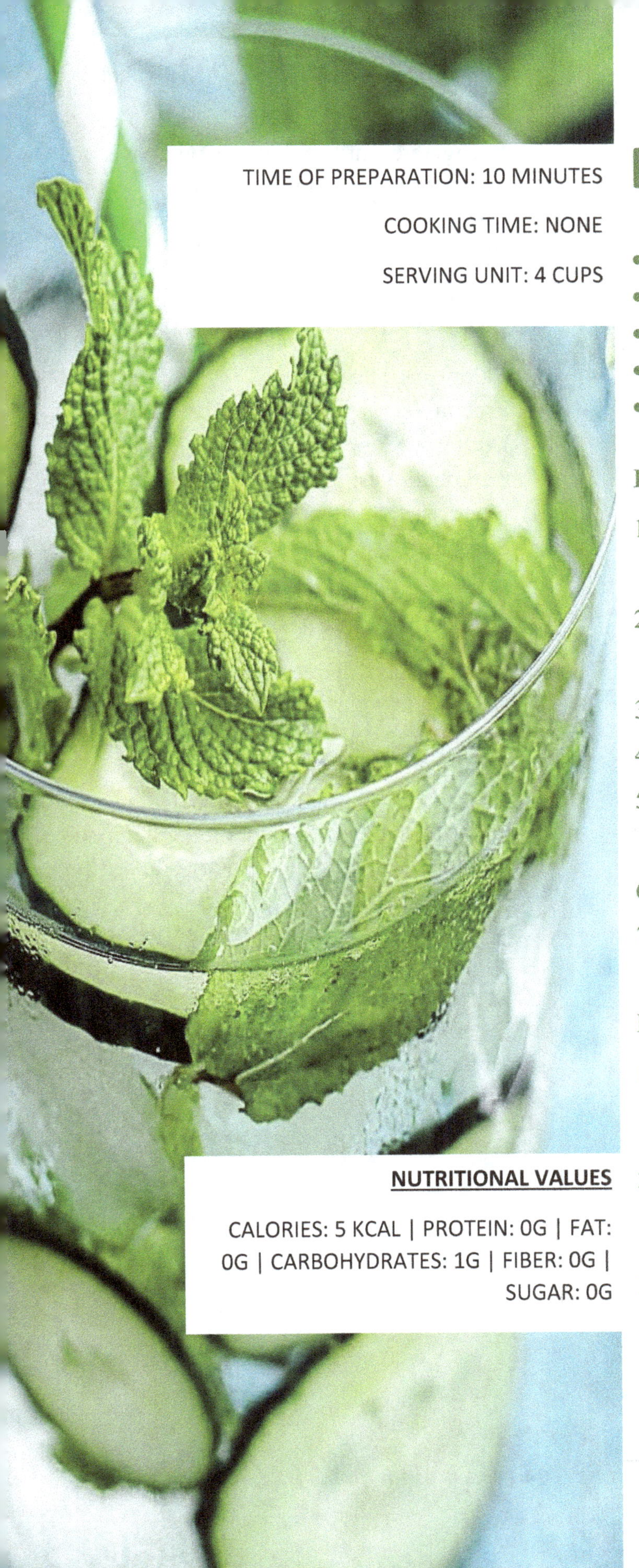

TIME OF PREPARATION: 10 MINUTES

COOKING TIME: NONE

SERVING UNIT: 4 CUPS

**NUTRITIONAL VALUES**

CALORIES: 5 KCAL | PROTEIN: 0G | FAT: 0G | CARBOHYDRATES: 1G | FIBER: 0G | SUGAR: 0G

# CUCUMBER MINT WATER

- 1 medium cucumber, thinly sliced
- 10 fresh mint leaves
- 4 cups cold water
- 1 lemon, thinly sliced (optional)
- Ice cubes (optional)

## PROCEDURES

1. Wash and thinly slice the cucumber and lemon (if using).
2. Place the cucumber slices, mint leaves, and lemon slices in a large pitcher.
3. Pour cold water over the ingredients.
4. Stir gently to combine.
5. Let the water infuse for at least 30 minutes in the refrigerator.
6. Add ice cubes just before serving if desired.
7. Serve chilled and enjoy.

## HEALTH BENEFITS

1. Hydration: Cucumber mint water is a refreshing way to increase your daily water intake, essential for overall health.
2. Detoxification: Cucumber and mint can aid in flushing out toxins and keeping the body clean and refreshed.
3. Low-calorie: This beverage is virtually calorie-free, making it an excellent choice for those monitoring their calorie intake.

# CITRUS GREEN TEA

**Time of Preparation:** 5 minutes

**Cooking Time:** 5 minutes

**Serving Unit:** 2 cups

## INGREDIENTS

- 2 green tea bags
- 2 cups water
- 1 lemon, sliced
- 1 lime, sliced
- 1 tablespoon honey or maple syrup (optional)
- Ice cubes (optional)
- Fresh mint leaves for garnish (optional)

## PROCEDURES

1. Bring 2 cups of water to a boil in a small saucepan.
2. Remove from heat and add the green tea bags.
3. Let the tea steep for 3-5 minutes, depending on desired strength.
4. Remove the tea bags and allow the tea to cool slightly.
5. In a pitcher, combine the brewed tea with sliced lemon and lime.
6. Stir in honey or maple syrup if using.
7. Refrigerate until chilled, or pour over ice cubes for immediate enjoyment.
8. Garnish with fresh mint leaves before serving if desired.

## NUTRITIONAL VALUES

- Calories: 10 kcal
- Protein: 0g
- Fat: 0g
- Carbohydrates: 3g
- Fiber: 1g
- Sugar: 2g

## HEALTH BENEFITS

1. Antioxidants: Green tea is rich in antioxidants, particularly catechins, which help protect cells from damage and reduce inflammation.
2. Vitamin C: Citrus fruits like lemon and lime are excellent sources of vitamin C, essential for immune function and skin health.
3. Hydration: Green tea and citrus water provide hydration while offering a flavorful alternative to plain water.
4. Digestive aid: Citrus fruits and green tea can aid in digestion and promote a healthy gut microbiome.

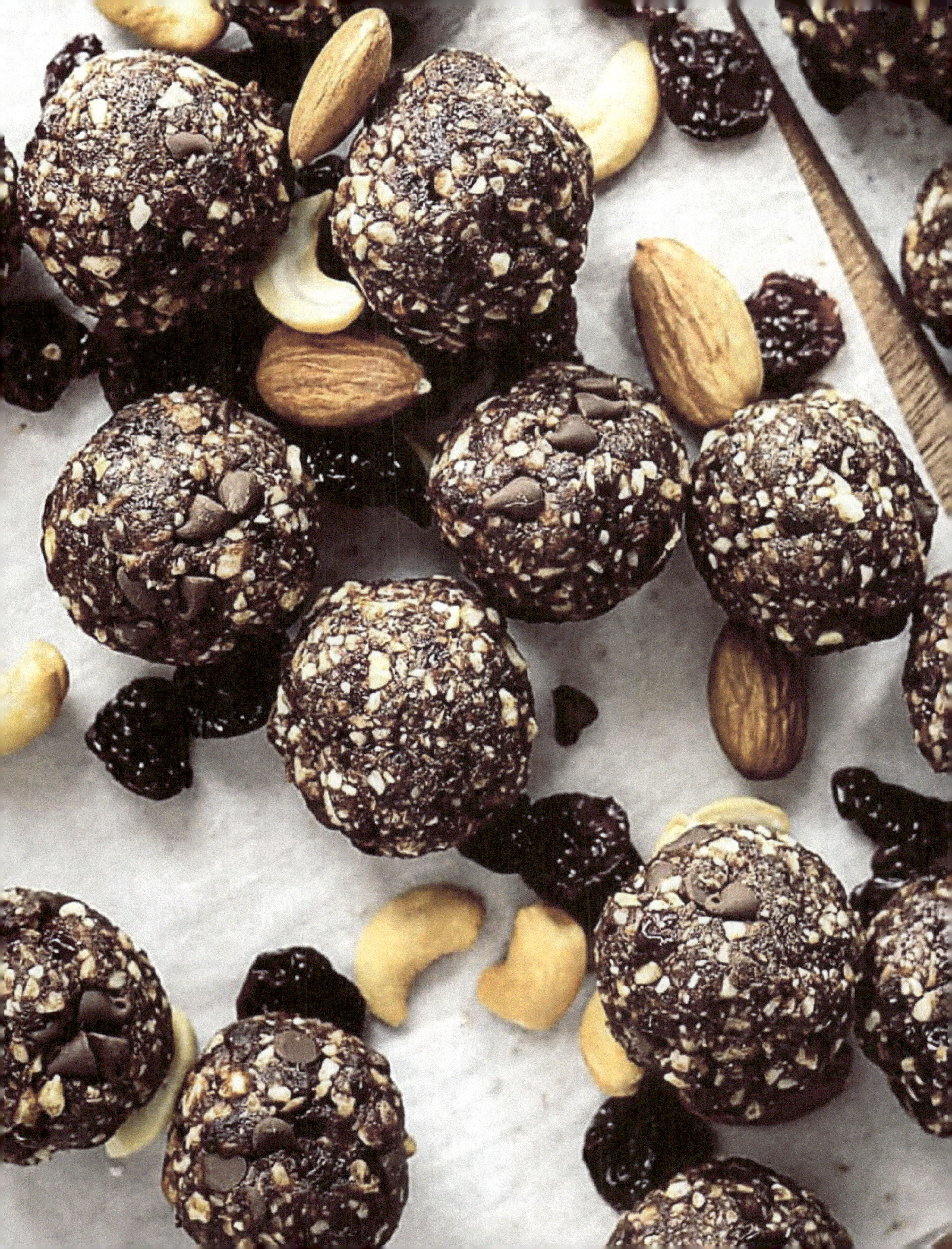

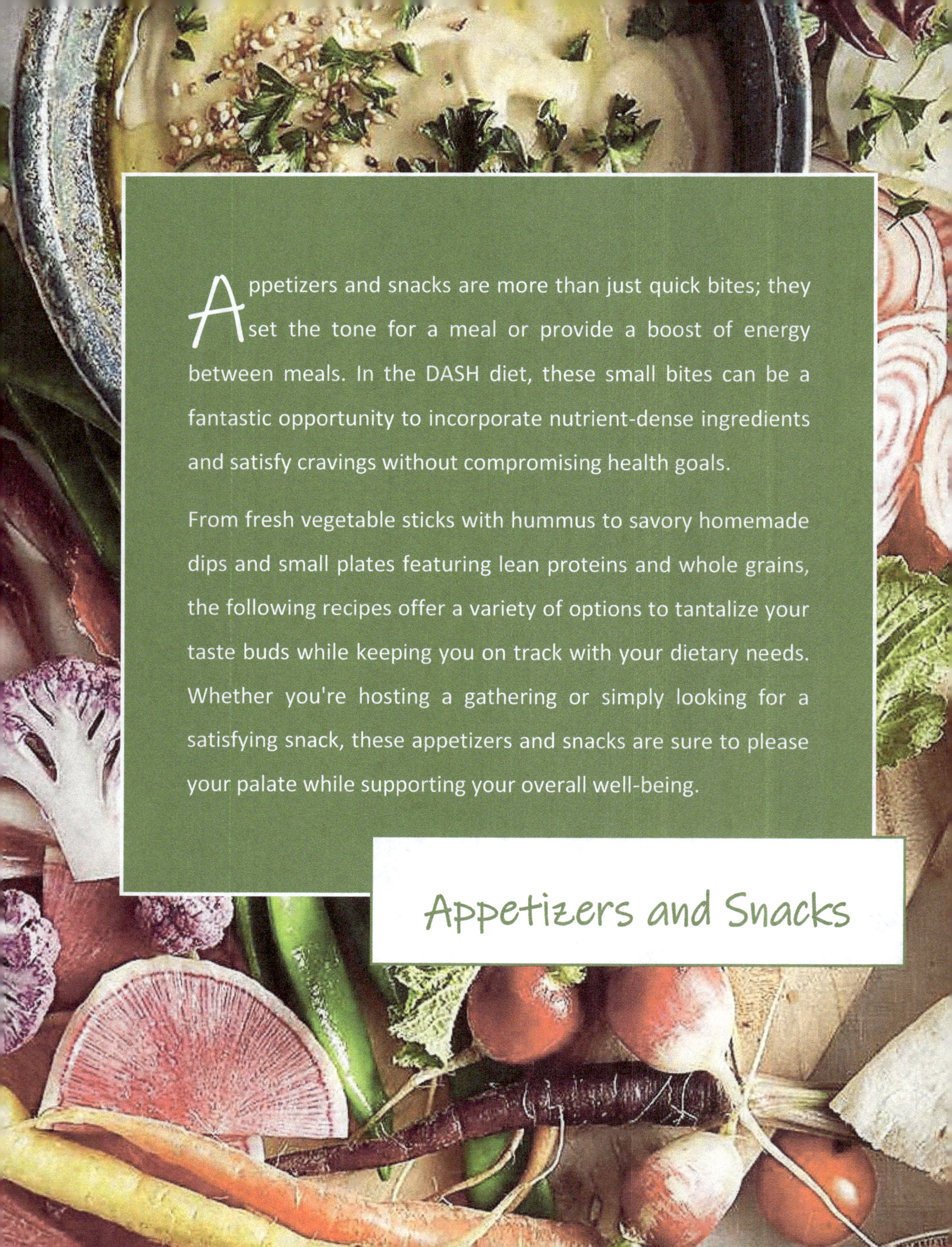

ppetizers and snacks are more than just quick bites; they set the tone for a meal or provide a boost of energy between meals. In the DASH diet, these small bites can be a fantastic opportunity to incorporate nutrient-dense ingredients and satisfy cravings without compromising health goals.

From fresh vegetable sticks with hummus to savory homemade dips and small plates featuring lean proteins and whole grains, the following recipes offer a variety of options to tantalize your taste buds while keeping you on track with your dietary needs. Whether you're hosting a gathering or simply looking for a satisfying snack, these appetizers and snacks are sure to please your palate while supporting your overall well-being.

## Appetizers and Snacks

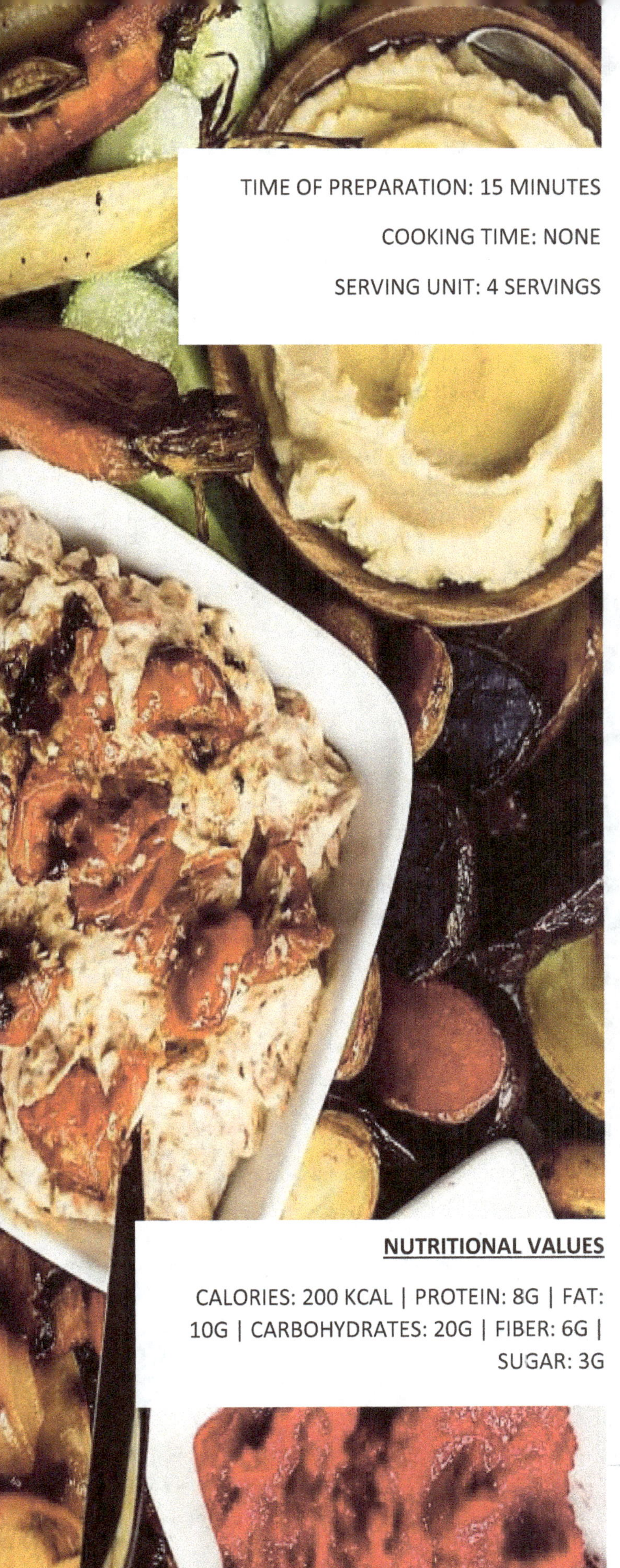

TIME OF PREPARATION: 15 MINUTES

COOKING TIME: NONE

SERVING UNIT: 4 SERVINGS

# HUMMUS AND VEGGIE PLATTER

- 1 cup hummus (store-bought or homemade)
- Assorted fresh vegetables (carrots, cucumbers, bell peppers, cherry tomatoes, celery)
- Whole grain pita bread or crackers

## PROCEDURES

1. Wash and prepare the vegetables by slicing them into sticks or bite-sized pieces.
2. Arrange the hummus in the center of a large platter or serving dish.
3. Surround the hummus with the assorted fresh vegetables.
4. Serve with whole grain pita bread or crackers on the side.
5. Enjoy dipping the vegetables and bread into the hummus for a nutritious and satisfying snack or appetizer.

## HEALTH BENEFITS

1. High in fiber: Both hummus and vegetables are rich in fiber, which supports digestion and helps you feel full.
2. Protein-packed: Hummus provides plant-based protein, which is important for muscle repair and growth.
3. Nutrient-dense: Vegetables are packed with vitamins, minerals, and antioxidants that support overall health and well-being.
4. Whole grain pita bread or crackers provide complex carbohydrates and fiber, contributing to heart health and stable blood sugar levels.

## NUTRITIONAL VALUES

CALORIES: 200 KCAL | PROTEIN: 8G | FAT: 10G | CARBOHYDRATES: 20G | FIBER: 6G | SUGAR: 3G

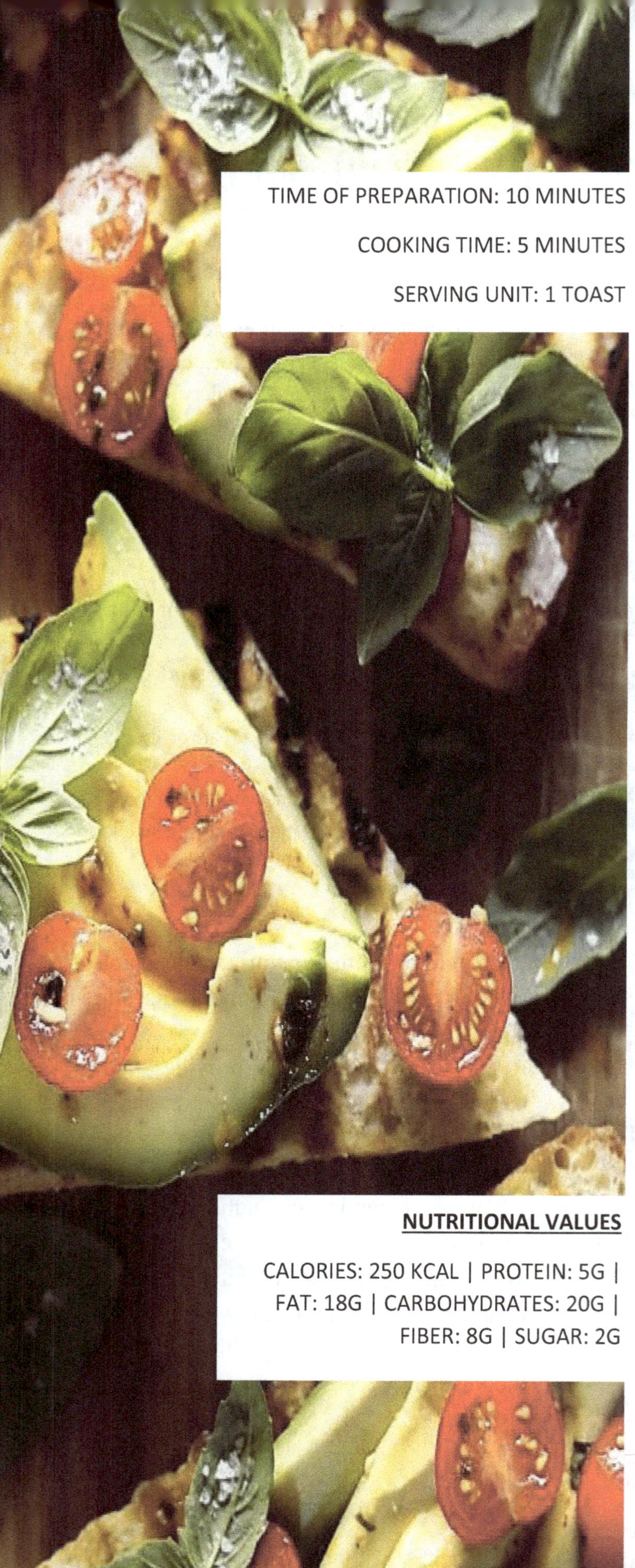

TIME OF PREPARATION: 10 MINUTES

COOKING TIME: 5 MINUTES

SERVING UNIT: 1 TOAST

## NUTRITIONAL VALUES

CALORIES: 250 KCAL | PROTEIN: 5G |
FAT: 18G | CARBOHYDRATES: 20G |
FIBER: 8G | SUGAR: 2G

# AVOCADO TOAST WITH TOMATO AND BASIL

- 1 slice whole grain bread
- 1/2 ripe avocado
- 1 small tomato, sliced
- 2-3 fresh basil leaves, chopped
- 1 teaspoon olive oil
- Salt and pepper to taste
- Optional: a squeeze of lemon juice, red pepper flakes for extra flavor

## PROCEDURES

1. Toast the slice of whole grain bread until golden brown and crispy.
2. While the bread is toasting, halve the avocado, remove the pit, and scoop the flesh into a bowl.
3. Mash the avocado with a fork until smooth, adding a pinch of salt and pepper to taste.
4. Spread the mashed avocado evenly onto the toasted bread.
5. Arrange the tomato slices on top of the avocado.
6. Drizzle with olive oil and sprinkle with chopped basil leaves.
7. Add a squeeze of lemon juice and red pepper flakes if desired.
8. Serve immediately and enjoy.

## HEALTH BENEFITS

1. Heart-healthy fats: Avocado is rich in monounsaturated fats, which are beneficial for heart health.
2. High in fiber: Whole grain bread and avocado provide fiber that aids digestion and keeps you feeling full longer.
3. Rich in vitamins and minerals: Tomatoes and avocados are packed with vitamins A, C, K, and potassium, supporting overall health.

# GREEK SALAD SKEWERS

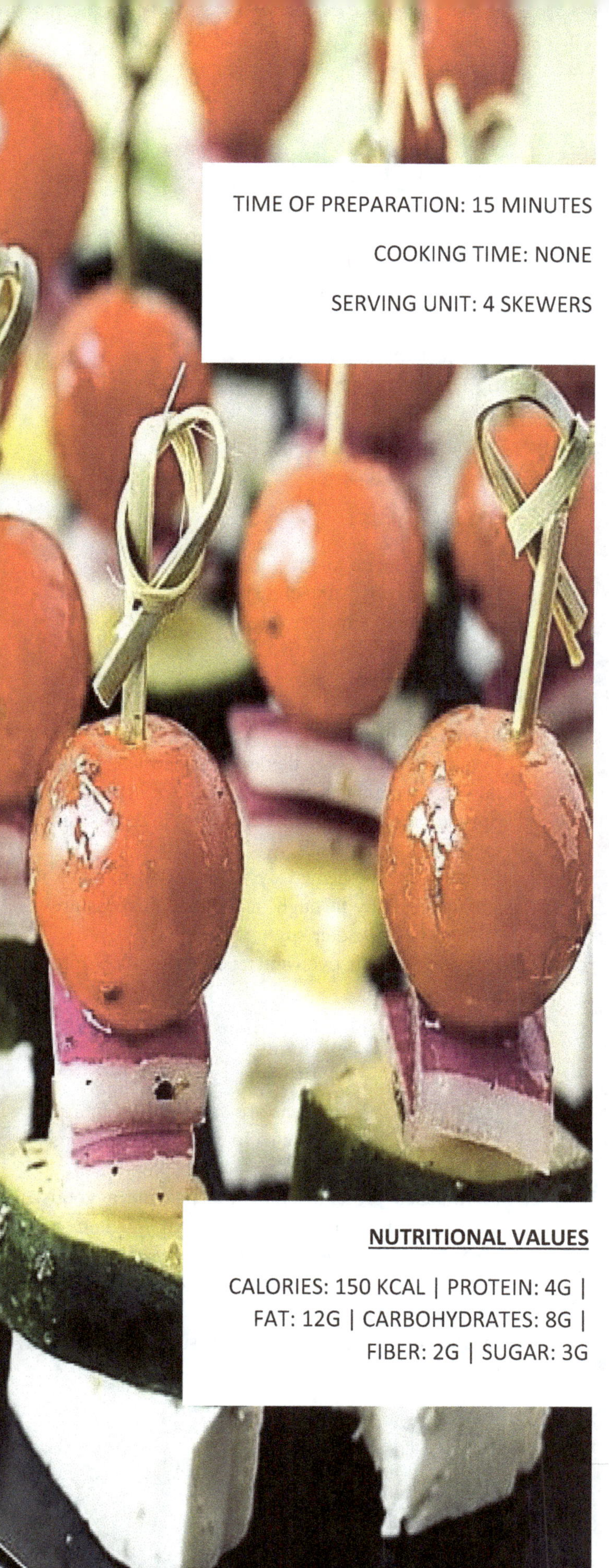

TIME OF PREPARATION: 15 MINUTES

COOKING TIME: NONE

SERVING UNIT: 4 SKEWERS

- 1 cup cherry tomatoes
- 1 cup cucumber, cut into thick slices
- 1/2 cup Kalamata olives, pitted
- 1/2 cup feta cheese, cut into cubes
- 1/2 small red onion, cut into chunks
- Fresh basil or mint leaves for garnish (optional)
- 1 tablespoon olive oil
- 1 teaspoon dried oregano
- Salt and pepper to taste
- Wooden or metal skewers

## PROCEDURES

1. Prepare the ingredients by washing the vegetables and cutting the cucumber, feta, and onion into bite-sized pieces.
2. Thread the cherry tomatoes, cucumber slices, Kalamata olives, feta cheese cubes, and red onion chunks alternately onto the skewers.
3. Arrange the skewers on a serving platter.
4. Drizzle olive oil over the skewers and sprinkle with dried oregano, salt, and pepper.
5. Garnish with fresh basil or mint leaves if desired.
6. Serve immediately or refrigerate until ready to serve.

## HEALTH BENEFITS

1. High in antioxidants: Tomatoes and cucumbers are rich in vitamins A and C, which protect cells from oxidative damage.
2. Heart-healthy fats: Olive oil and olives provide monounsaturated fats that are beneficial for heart health.
3. Low in calories: This light and refreshing appetizer is low in calories but packed with nutrients, making it a great option for weight management.

## NUTRITIONAL VALUES

CALORIES: 150 KCAL | PROTEIN: 4G | FAT: 12G | CARBOHYDRATES: 8G | FIBER: 2G | SUGAR: 3G

# ROASTED CHICKPEAS

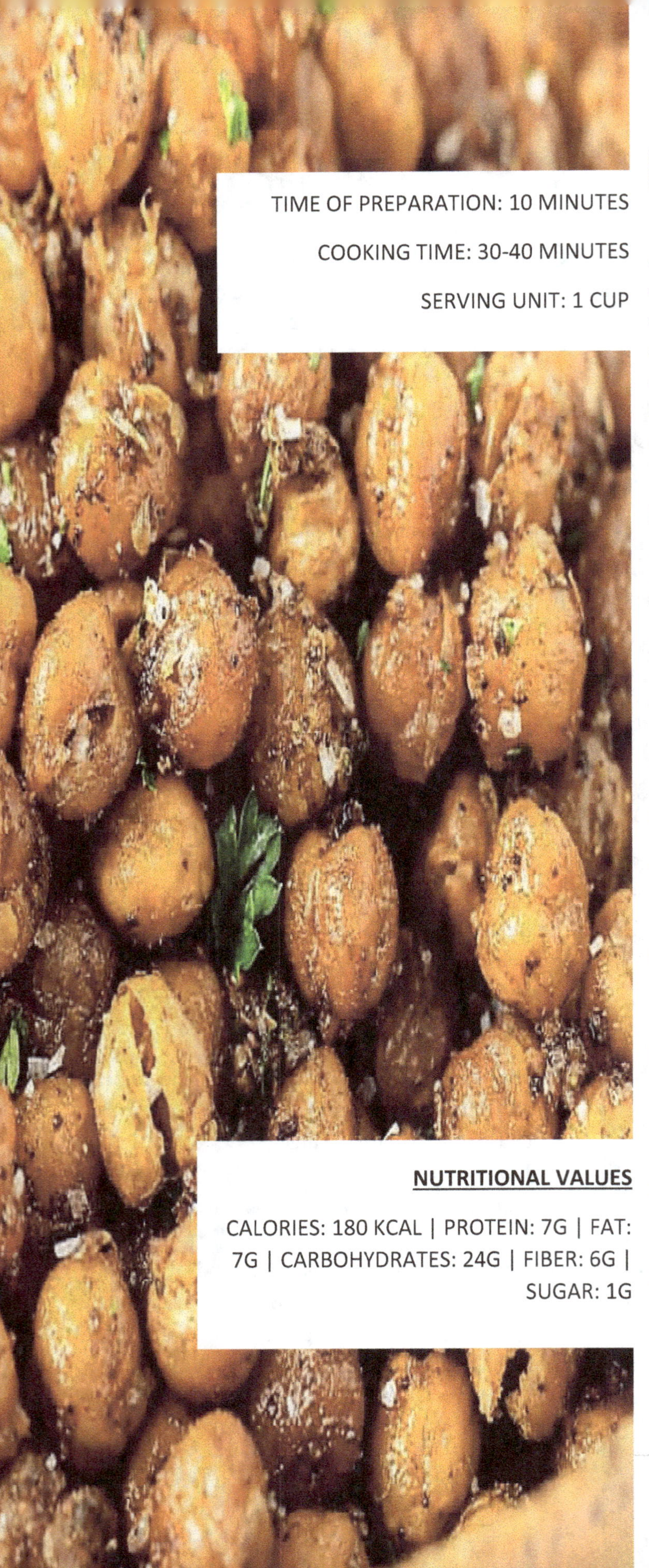

TIME OF PREPARATION: 10 MINUTES

COOKING TIME: 30-40 MINUTES

SERVING UNIT: 1 CUP

- 1 can (15 oz) chickpeas, drained and rinsed
- 1 tablespoon olive oil
- 1 teaspoon smoked paprika
- 1/2 teaspoon garlic powder
- 1/2 teaspoon ground cumin
- 1/2 teaspoon salt
- 1/4 teaspoon black pepper

## PROCEDURES

1. Preheat the oven to 400°F (200°C).
2. Drain and rinse the chickpeas thoroughly. Pat them dry with paper towels.
3. Spread the chickpeas on a baking sheet lined with parchment paper.
4. Drizzle the olive oil over the chickpeas and toss to coat evenly.
5. In a small bowl, mix the smoked paprika, garlic powder, ground cumin, salt, and black pepper.
6. Sprinkle the spice mixture over the chickpeas and toss again to coat evenly.
7. Roast in the preheated oven for 30-40 minutes, stirring halfway through, until the chickpeas are golden brown and crispy.
8. Remove from the oven and let cool slightly before serving.

## HEALTH BENEFITS

1. High in fiber: Chickpeas are an excellent source of dietary fiber, which aids in digestion and helps maintain a healthy weight.
2. Plant-based protein: Chickpeas provide a good amount of plant-based protein, making them a great snack for vegetarians and vegans.
3. Rich in vitamins and minerals: Chickpeas contain important nutrients such as folate, iron, magnesium, and zinc, which support overall health.

### NUTRITIONAL VALUES

CALORIES: 180 KCAL | PROTEIN: 7G | FAT: 7G | CARBOHYDRATES: 24G | FIBER: 6G | SUGAR: 1G

# FRUIT AND NUT ENERGY BITES

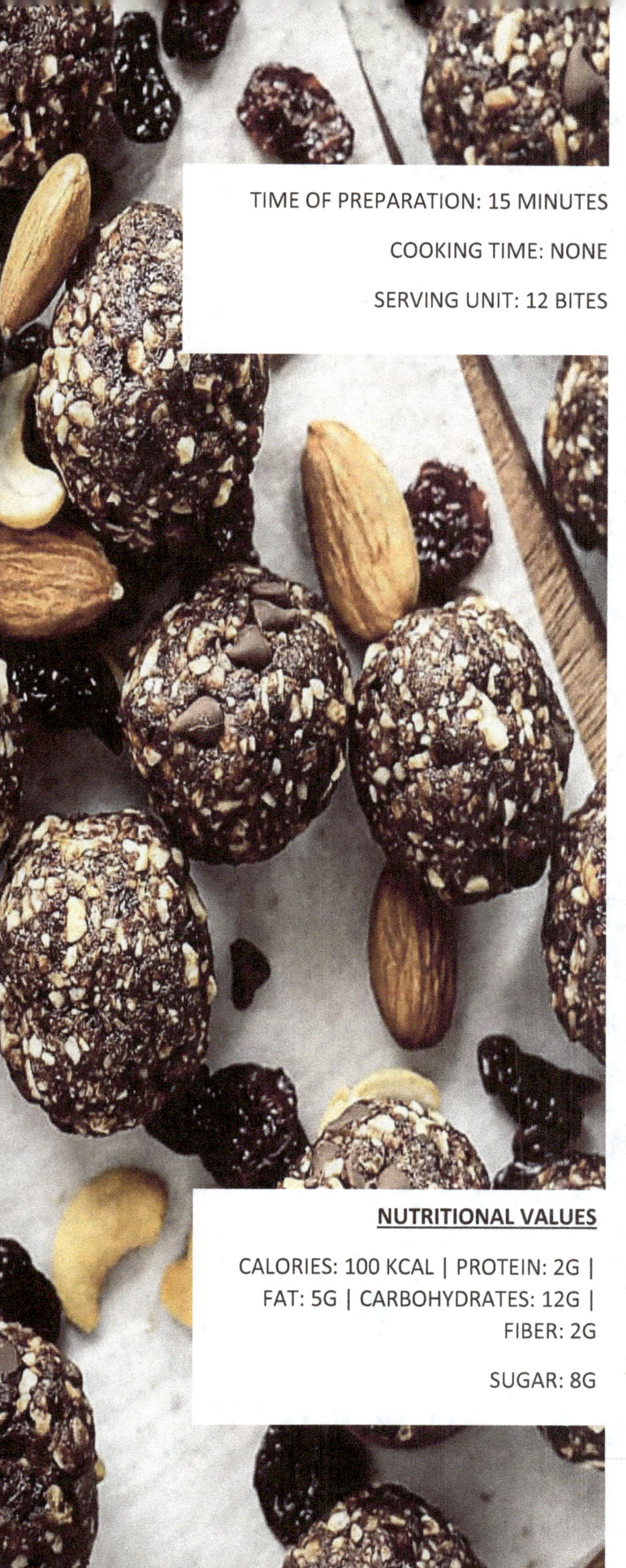

TIME OF PREPARATION: 15 MINUTES

COOKING TIME: NONE

SERVING UNIT: 12 BITES

- 1 cup pitted dates
- 1/2 cup raw almonds
- 1/2 cup raw cashews
- 1/4 cup unsweetened shredded coconut
- 1/4 cup dried cranberries or raisins
- 1 tablespoon chia seeds or flaxseeds
- 1 tablespoon honey or maple syrup (optional)
- 1/2 teaspoon vanilla extract
- Pinch of salt

## PROCEDURES

1. Place the dates in a food processor and blend until they form a sticky paste.
2. Add the almonds, cashews, shredded coconut, dried cranberries or raisins, chia seeds or flaxseeds, honey or maple syrup, vanilla extract, and salt.
3. Pulse the mixture until it is well combined and forms a sticky dough.
4. Scoop out tablespoon-sized portions of the mixture and roll into balls.
5. Place the energy bites on a baking sheet lined with parchment paper.
6. Refrigerate for at least 30 minutes to firm up.
7. Store in an airtight container in the refrigerator for up to 1 week or in the freezer for up to 3 months.

## HEALTH BENEFITS

1. Energy boost: Dates and dried fruits provide natural sugars and carbohydrates for a quick energy boost.
2. High in fiber: Nuts and seeds contribute to the fiber content, promoting digestive health and satiety.
3. Healthy fats: Almonds and cashews offer heart-healthy monounsaturated fats and essential fatty acids.

### NUTRITIONAL VALUES

CALORIES: 100 KCAL | PROTEIN: 2G | FAT: 5G | CARBOHYDRATES: 12G | FIBER: 2G

SUGAR: 8G

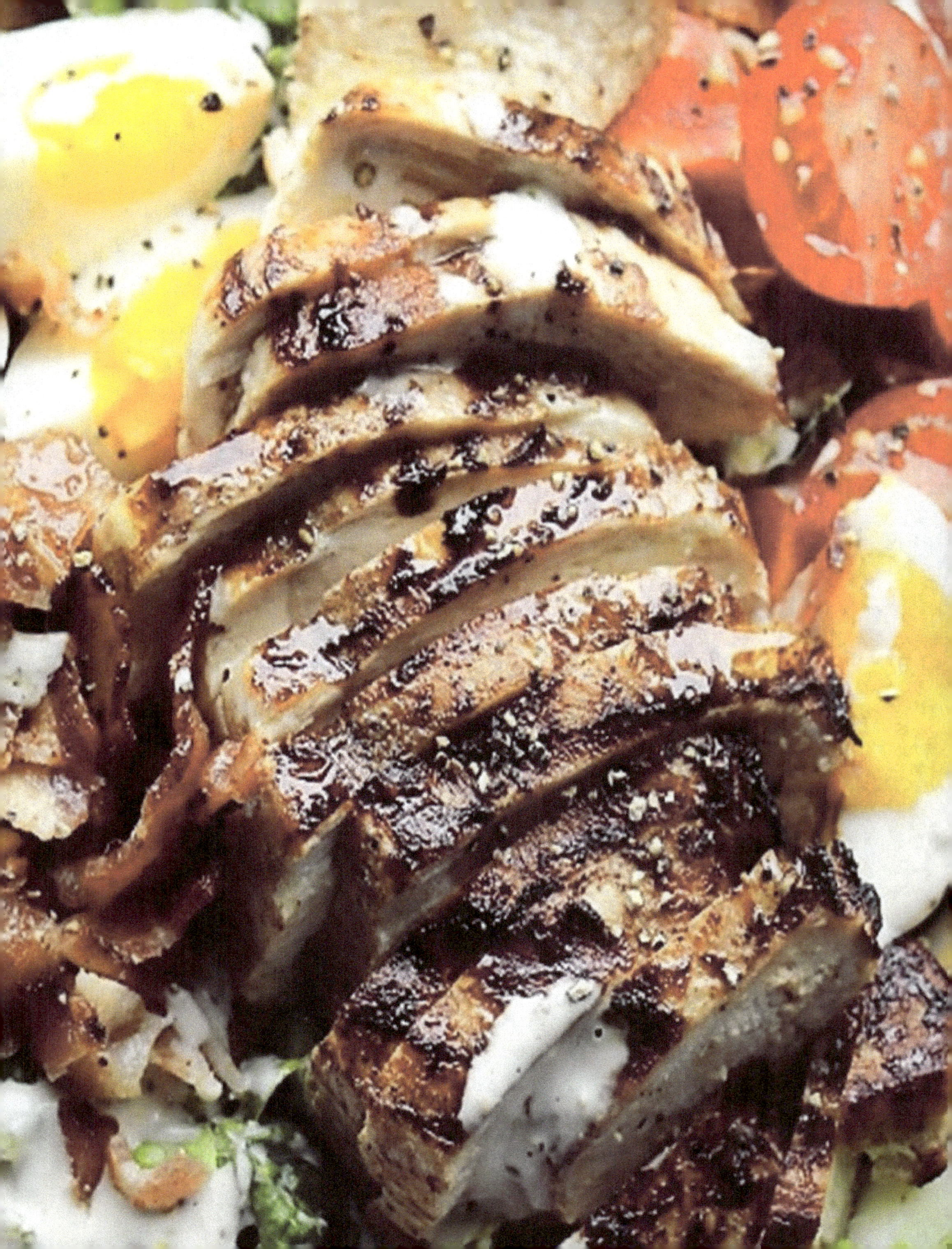

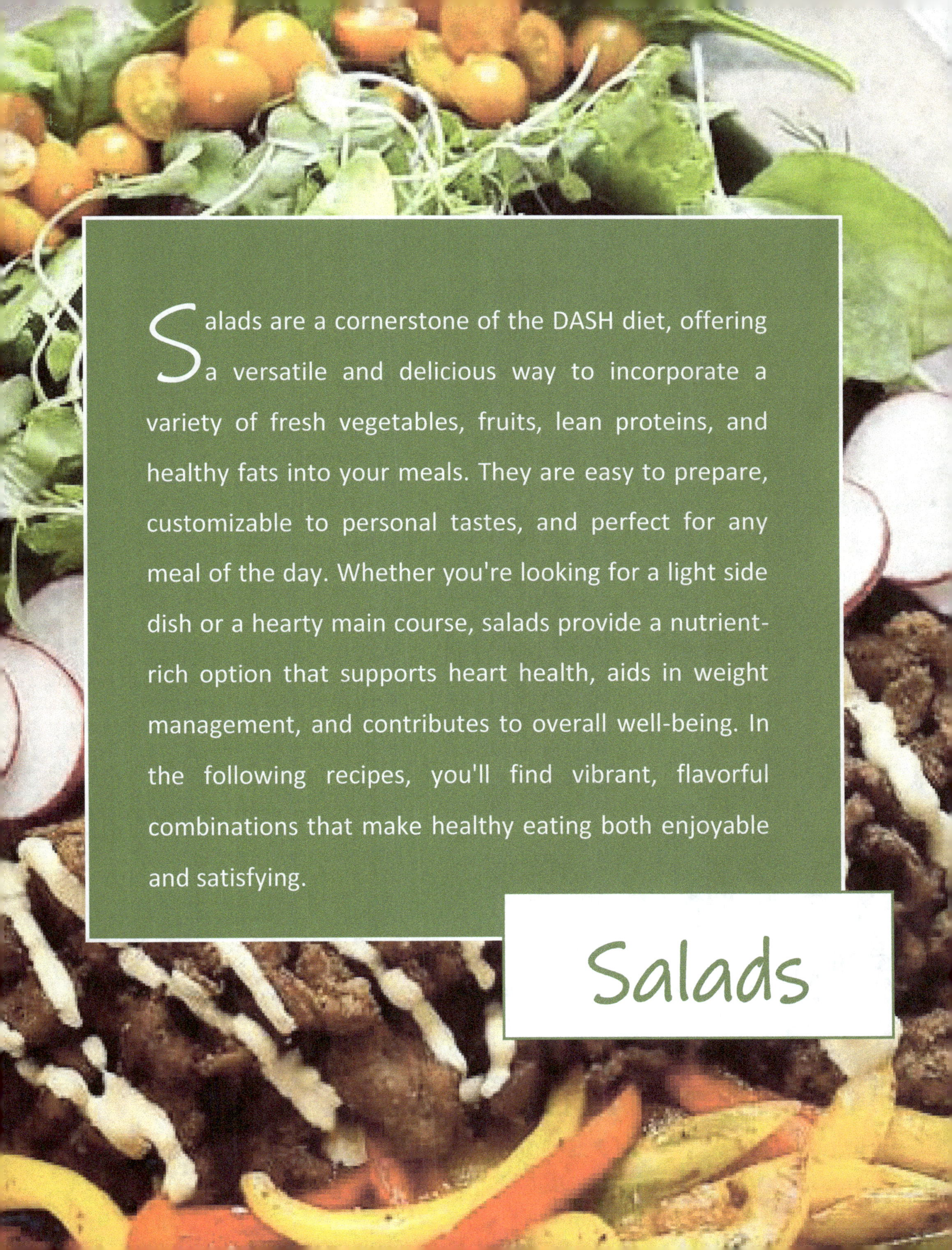


Salads are a cornerstone of the DASH diet, offering a versatile and delicious way to incorporate a variety of fresh vegetables, fruits, lean proteins, and healthy fats into your meals. They are easy to prepare, customizable to personal tastes, and perfect for any meal of the day. Whether you're looking for a light side dish or a hearty main course, salads provide a nutrient-rich option that supports heart health, aids in weight management, and contributes to overall well-being. In the following recipes, you'll find vibrant, flavorful combinations that make healthy eating both enjoyable and satisfying.

Salads

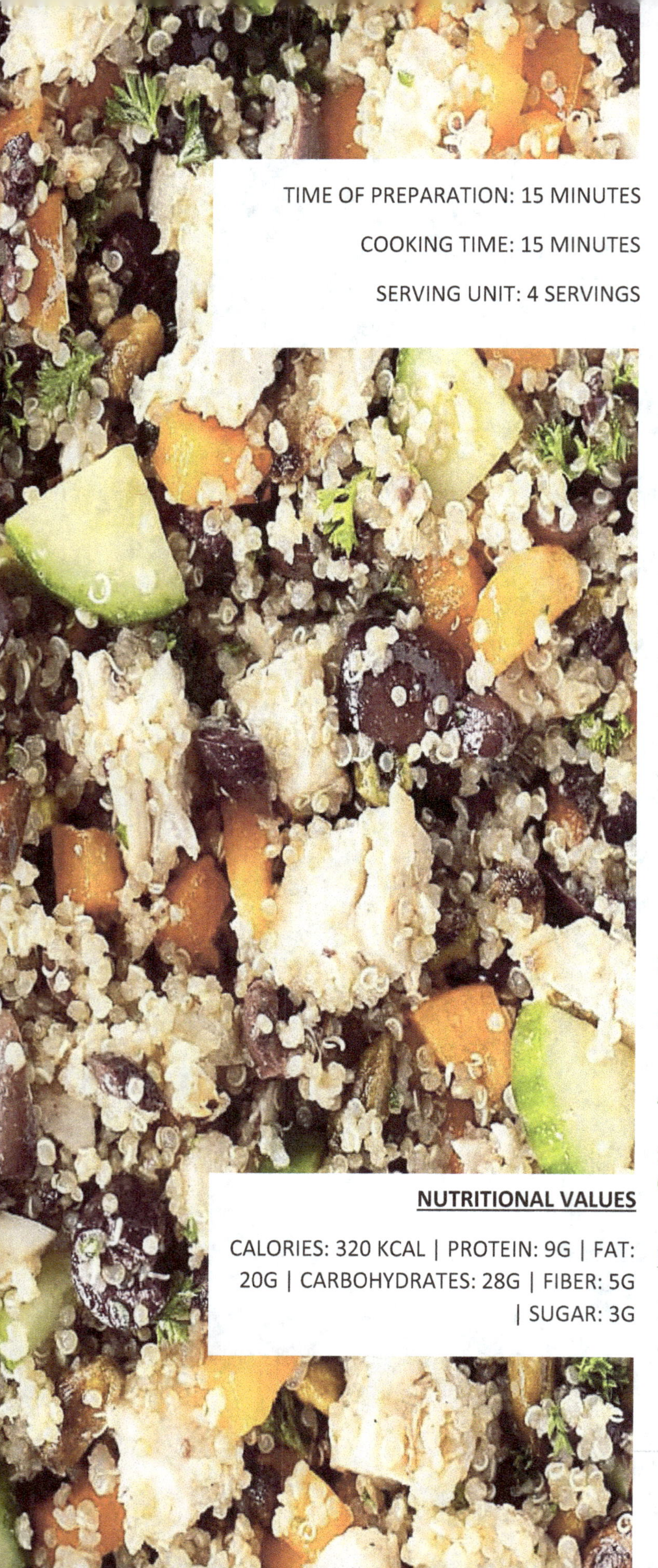

TIME OF PREPARATION: 15 MINUTES

COOKING TIME: 15 MINUTES

SERVING UNIT: 4 SERVINGS

# MEDITERRANEAN QUINOA SALAD

- 1 cup quinoa
- 2 cups water or vegetable broth
- 1 cup cherry tomatoes, halved
- 1 cup cucumber, diced
- 1/2 cup Kalamata olives, pitted and sliced
- 1/2 cup feta cheese, crumbled
- 1/4 cup red onion, finely chopped
- 1/4 cup fresh parsley, chopped
- 1/4 cup fresh mint, chopped
- 1/4 cup olive oil
- 2 tablespoons lemon juice
- 1 teaspoon dried oregano
- Salt and pepper to taste

## PROCEDURES

1. Rinse the quinoa under cold water. In a medium saucepan, bring the water or vegetable broth to a boil. Add the quinoa, reduce heat to low, cover, and simmer for 15 minutes, or until the quinoa is tender and the liquid is absorbed.
2. Remove the quinoa from heat and let it cool to room temperature.
3. In a large bowl, combine the cooked quinoa, cherry tomatoes, cucumber, olives, feta cheese, red onion, parsley, and mint.
4. In a small bowl, whisk together the olive oil, lemon juice, dried oregano, salt, and pepper.
5. Pour the dressing over the salad and toss to combine.
6. Adjust seasoning to taste and serve immediately or refrigerate until ready to serve.

## HEALTH BENEFITS

1. High in fiber: Quinoa and vegetables provide dietary fiber, which aids digestion and helps you feel full longer.

## NUTRITIONAL VALUES

CALORIES: 320 KCAL | PROTEIN: 9G | FAT: 20G | CARBOHYDRATES: 28G | FIBER: 5G | SUGAR: 3G

# KALE AND APPLE SALAD WITH WALNUTS

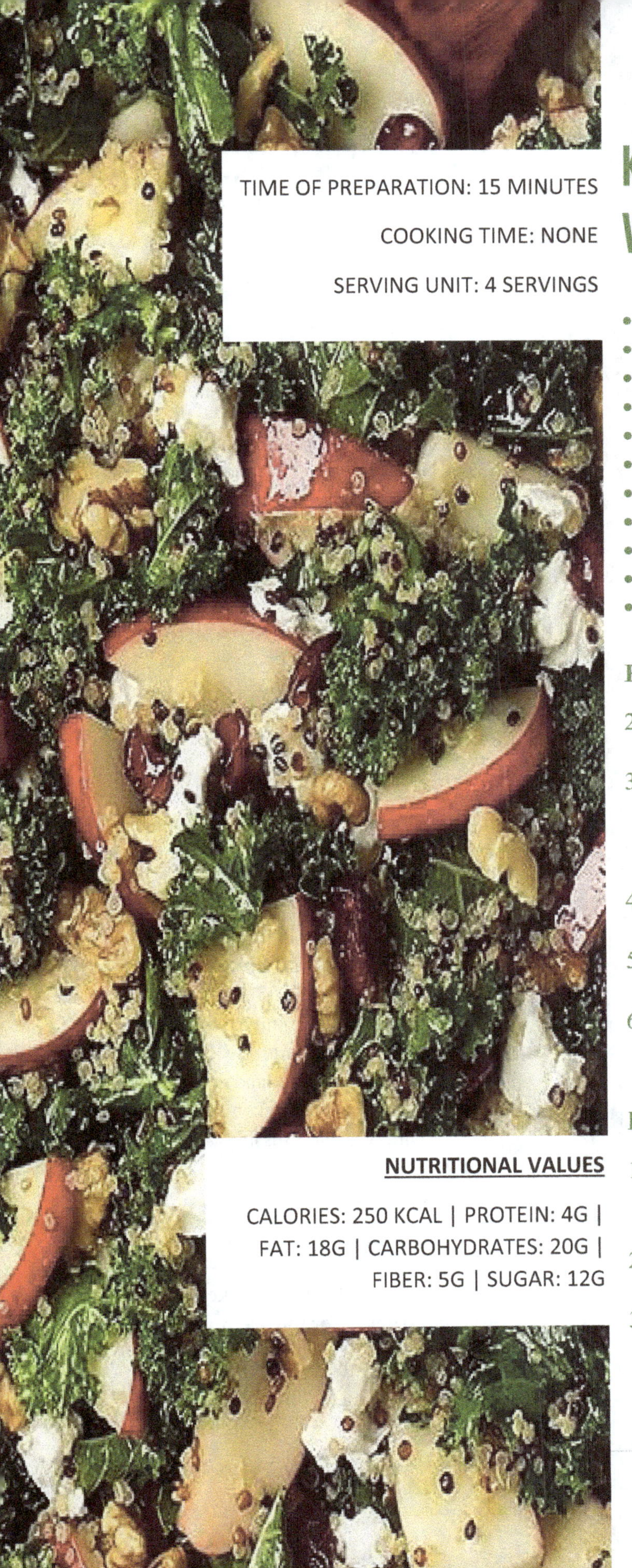

TIME OF PREPARATION: 15 MINUTES

COOKING TIME: NONE

SERVING UNIT: 4 SERVINGS

- 6 cups kale, de-stemmed and chopped
- 1 large apple, thinly sliced
- 1/2 cup walnuts, toasted and chopped
- 1/4 cup dried cranberries
- 1/4 cup red onion, thinly sliced
- 1/4 cup feta cheese, crumbled (optional)
- 3 tablespoons olive oil
- 1 tablespoon apple cider vinegar
- 1 tablespoon honey or maple syrup
- 1 teaspoon Dijon mustard
- Salt and pepper to taste

## PROCEDURES

2. In a large bowl, combine the kale, apple slices, walnuts, dried cranberries, and red onion.
3. In a small bowl, whisk together the olive oil, apple cider vinegar, honey or maple syrup, Dijon mustard, salt, and pepper until well combined.
4. Pour the dressing over the salad and toss to coat the ingredients evenly.
5. If desired, sprinkle the salad with feta cheese before serving.
6. Serve immediately or refrigerate until ready to serve.

## HEALTH BENEFITS

1. Nutrient-dense: Kale is rich in vitamins A, C, and K, as well as minerals like calcium and potassium, which support overall health.
2. High in fiber: Kale, apples, and walnuts provide dietary fiber, promoting digestion and satiety.
3. Heart-healthy fats: Walnuts and olive oil add monounsaturated fats and omega-3 fatty acids, beneficial for heart health.

### NUTRITIONAL VALUES

CALORIES: 250 KCAL | PROTEIN: 4G | FAT: 18G | CARBOHYDRATES: 20G | FIBER: 5G | SUGAR: 12G

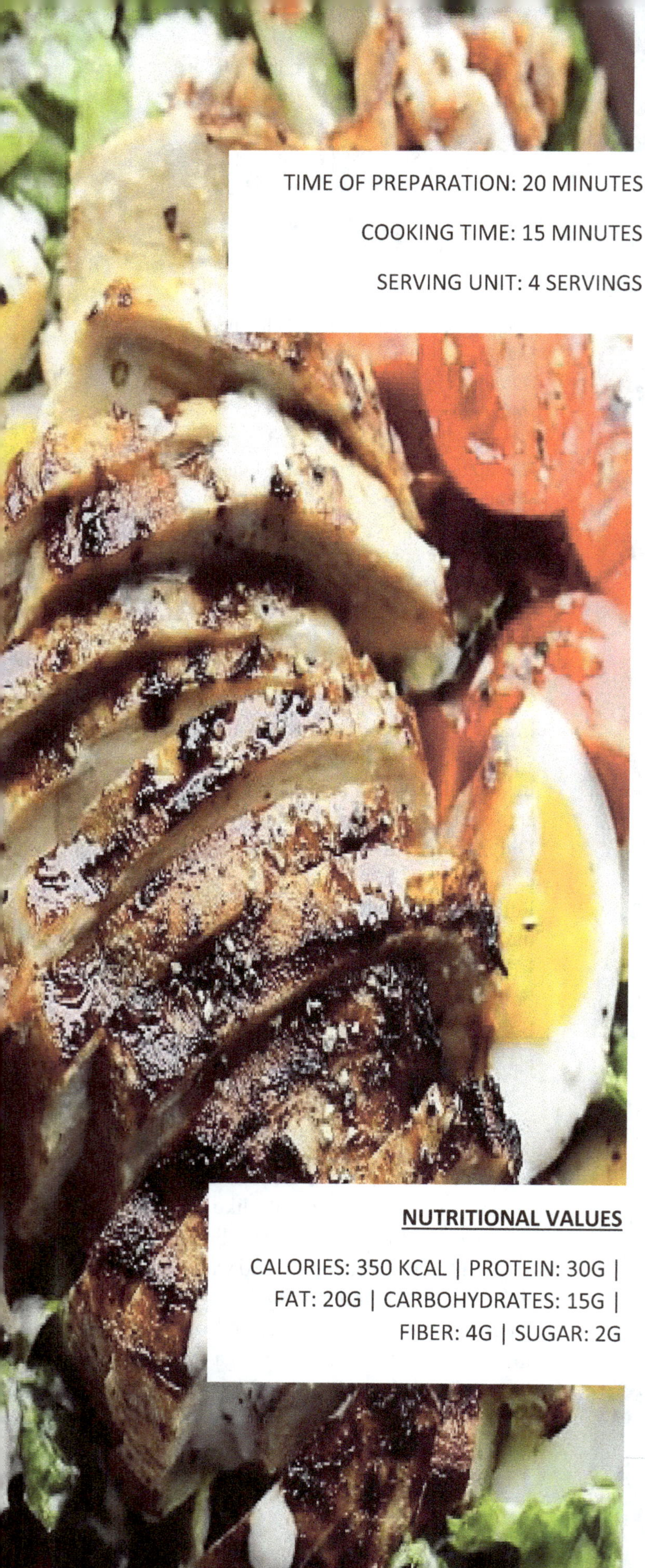

TIME OF PREPARATION: 20 MINUTES

COOKING TIME: 15 MINUTES

SERVING UNIT: 4 SERVINGS

**NUTRITIONAL VALUES**

CALORIES: 350 KCAL | PROTEIN: 30G |
FAT: 20G | CARBOHYDRATES: 15G |
FIBER: 4G | SUGAR: 2G

# GRILLED CHICKEN CAESAR SALAD

- 2 boneless, skinless chicken breasts
- 6 cups romaine lettuce, chopped
- 1/2 cup Parmesan cheese, shaved
- 1 cup whole grain croutons
- 1/4 cup Caesar dressing (store-bought or homemade)

### *Marinade for Chicken:*

- 2 tablespoons olive oil
- 1 tablespoon lemon juice
- 1 teaspoon garlic powder
- Salt and pepper to taste

## PROCEDURES

1. Preheat the grill to medium-high heat.
2. In a bowl, mix olive oil, lemon juice, garlic powder, salt, and pepper to make the marinade. Coat the chicken breasts with the marinade and let sit for 10-15 minutes.
3. Grill the chicken breasts for 6-7 minutes on each side or until fully cooked and the internal temperature reaches 165°F (74°C). Let the chicken rest for a few minutes, then slice.
4. In a large bowl, combine the chopped romaine lettuce, Parmesan cheese, and croutons.
5. Add the sliced grilled chicken to the salad.
6. Drizzle with Caesar dressing and toss to coat evenly.
7. Serve immediately.

## HEALTH BENEFITS

1. High in protein: Grilled chicken provides lean protein, essential for muscle repair and growth.
2. Low in carbohydrates: This salad is low in carbs, making it suitable for low-carb diets.

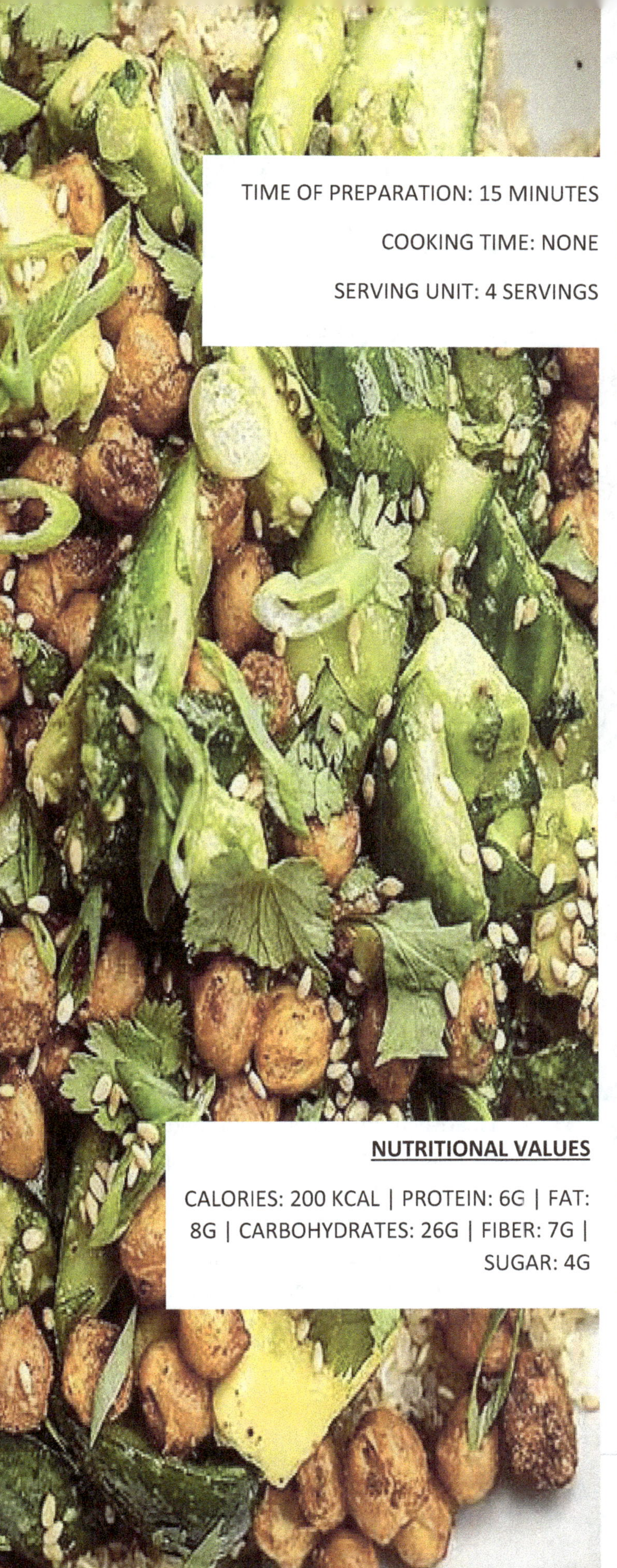

TIME OF PREPARATION: 15 MINUTES

COOKING TIME: NONE

SERVING UNIT: 4 SERVINGS

**NUTRITIONAL VALUES**

CALORIES: 200 KCAL | PROTEIN: 6G | FAT: 8G | CARBOHYDRATES: 26G | FIBER: 7G | SUGAR: 4G

# CHICKPEA AND CUCUMBER SALAD

- 1 can (15 oz) chickpeas, drained and rinsed
- 1 cucumber, diced
- 1 bell pepper, diced
- 1/4 red onion, thinly sliced
- 1/4 cup fresh parsley, chopped
- 2 tablespoons olive oil
- 2 tablespoons lemon juice
- 1 teaspoon dried oregano
- Salt and pepper to taste

## PROCEDURES

1. In a large bowl, combine the chickpeas, diced cucumber, diced bell pepper, sliced red onion, and chopped parsley.
2. In a small bowl, whisk together the olive oil, lemon juice, dried oregano, salt, and pepper.
3. Pour the dressing over the salad and toss to coat the ingredients evenly.
4. Adjust seasoning to taste and serve immediately or refrigerate until ready to serve.

## HEALTH BENEFITS

1. High in fiber: Chickpeas and vegetables provide dietary fiber, promoting digestive health and keeping you full longer.
2. Plant-based protein: Chickpeas are a good source of protein, making this salad a satisfying vegetarian option.
3. Low in calories: This salad is low in calories but high in nutrients, making it a great choice for weight management.

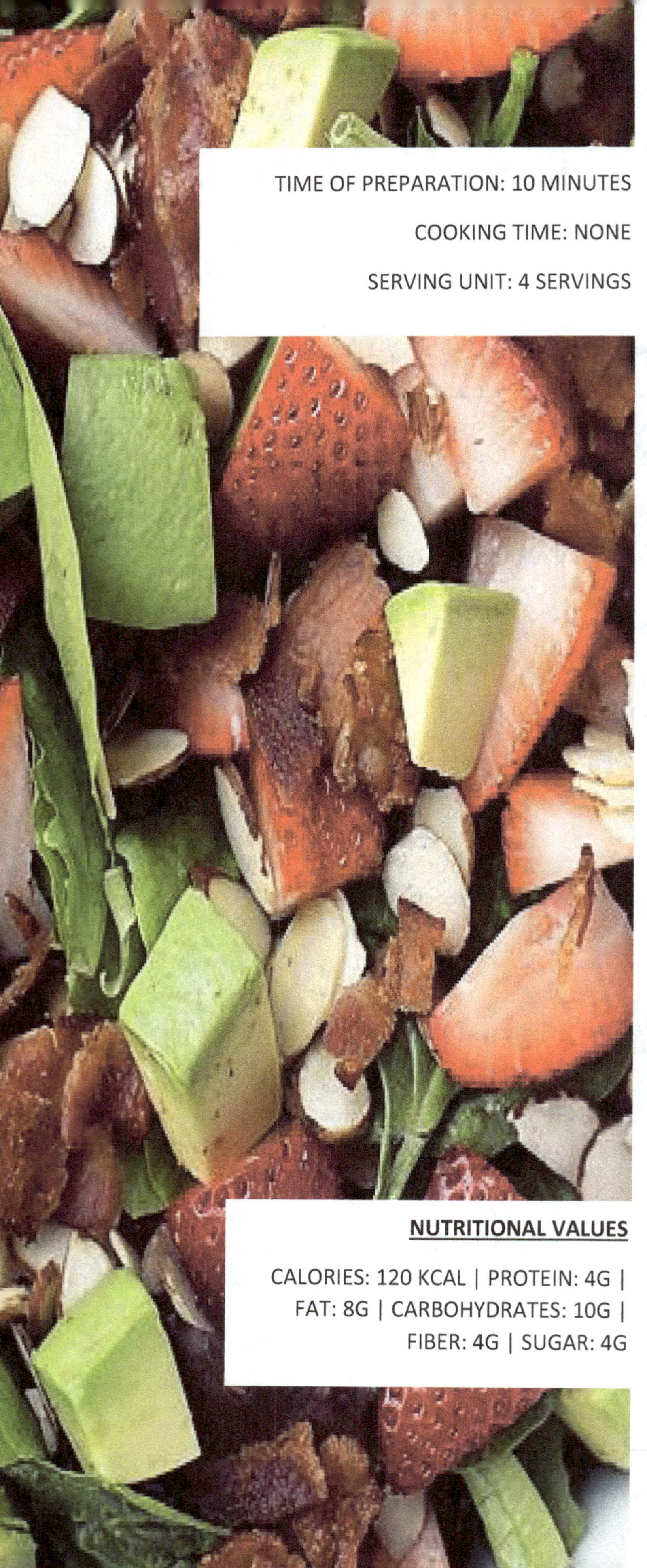



# SPINACH, STRAWBERRY, AND ALMOND SALAD

TIME OF PREPARATION: 10 MINUTES

COOKING TIME: NONE

SERVING UNIT: 4 SERVINGS

- 6 cups baby spinach leaves
- 1 cup strawberries, sliced
- 1/4 cup sliced almonds, toasted
- 1/4 cup crumbled feta cheese (optional)
- Balsamic vinaigrette dressing

## PROCEDURES

1. In a large bowl, combine the baby spinach leaves, sliced strawberries, toasted sliced almonds, and crumbled feta cheese.
2. Drizzle with balsamic vinaigrette dressing and toss gently to coat the ingredients evenly.
3. Serve immediately.

## HEALTH BENEFITS

1. Nutrient-dense: Spinach is rich in vitamins A, C, and K, as well as iron, magnesium, and potassium.
2. Antioxidants: Strawberries are packed with antioxidants like vitamin C, which help protect cells from damage and boost immune function.
3. Heart-healthy fats: Almonds provide monounsaturated fats that support heart health and satiety.
4. Low in calories: This salad is low in calories but high in nutrients, making it an ideal option for weight management.

### NUTRITIONAL VALUES

CALORIES: 120 KCAL | PROTEIN: 4G | FAT: 8G | CARBOHYDRATES: 10G | FIBER: 4G | SUGAR: 4G

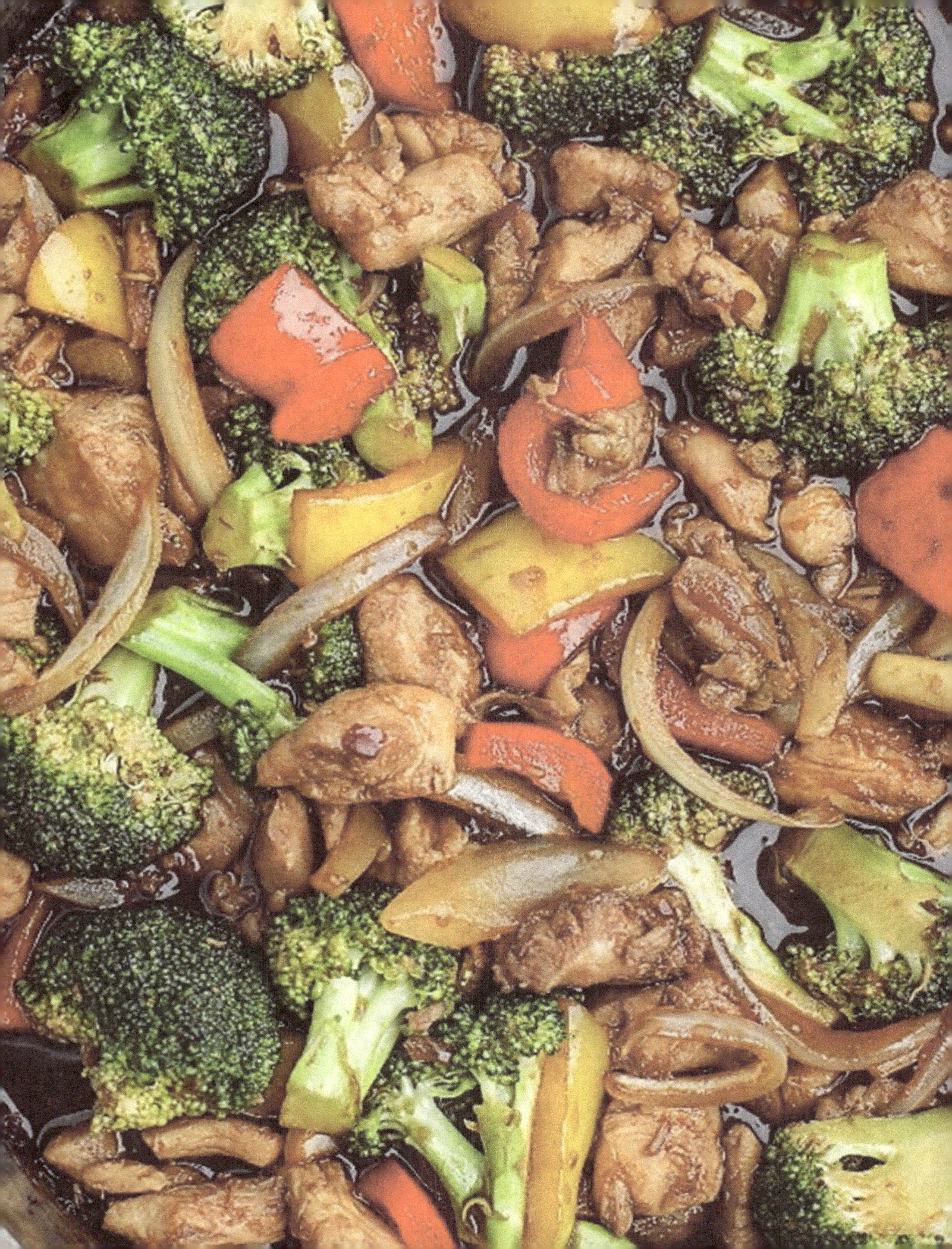

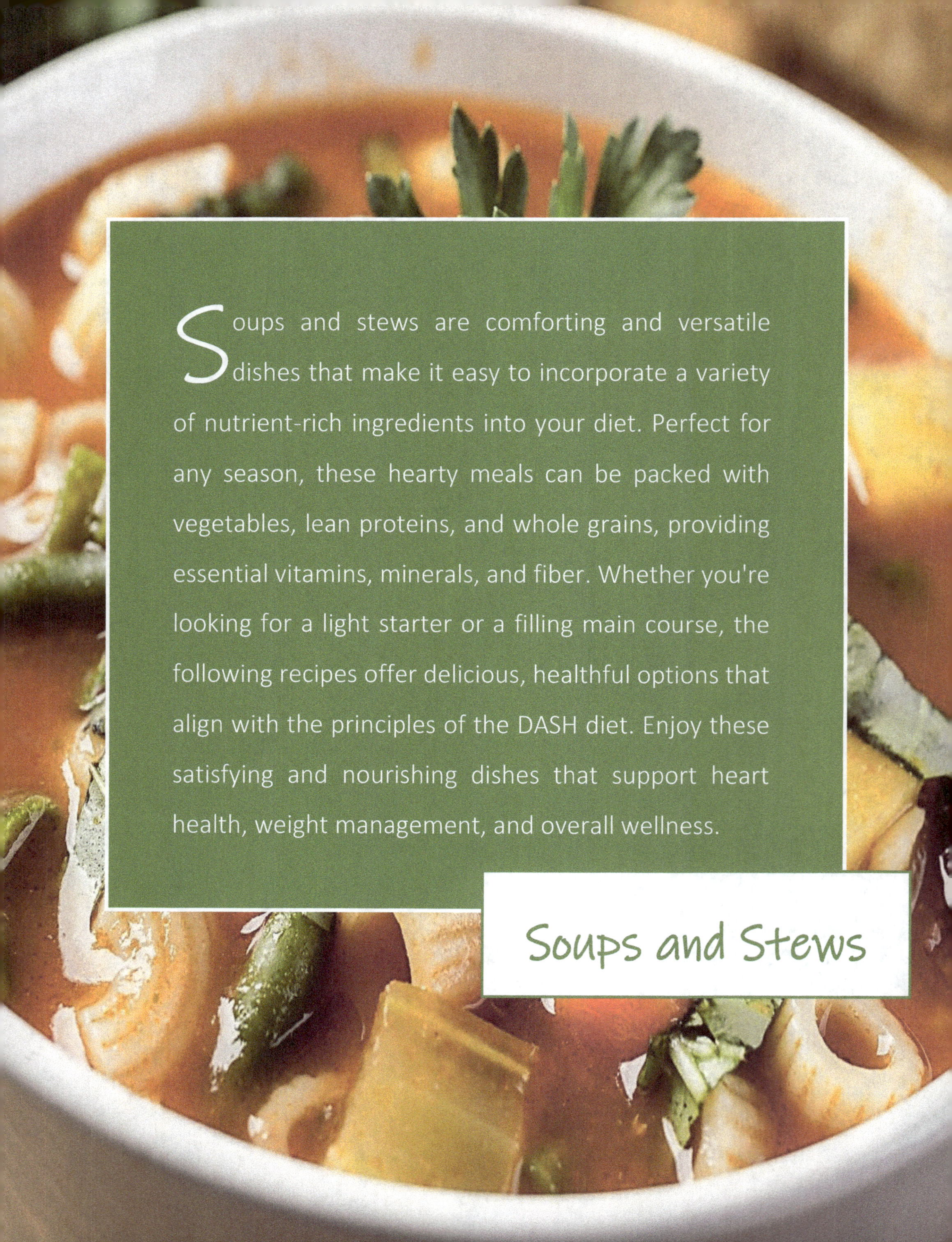
Soups and stews are comforting and versatile dishes that make it easy to incorporate a variety of nutrient-rich ingredients into your diet. Perfect for any season, these hearty meals can be packed with vegetables, lean proteins, and whole grains, providing essential vitamins, minerals, and fiber. Whether you're looking for a light starter or a filling main course, the following recipes offer delicious, healthful options that align with the principles of the DASH diet. Enjoy these satisfying and nourishing dishes that support heart health, weight management, and overall wellness.

Soups and Stews

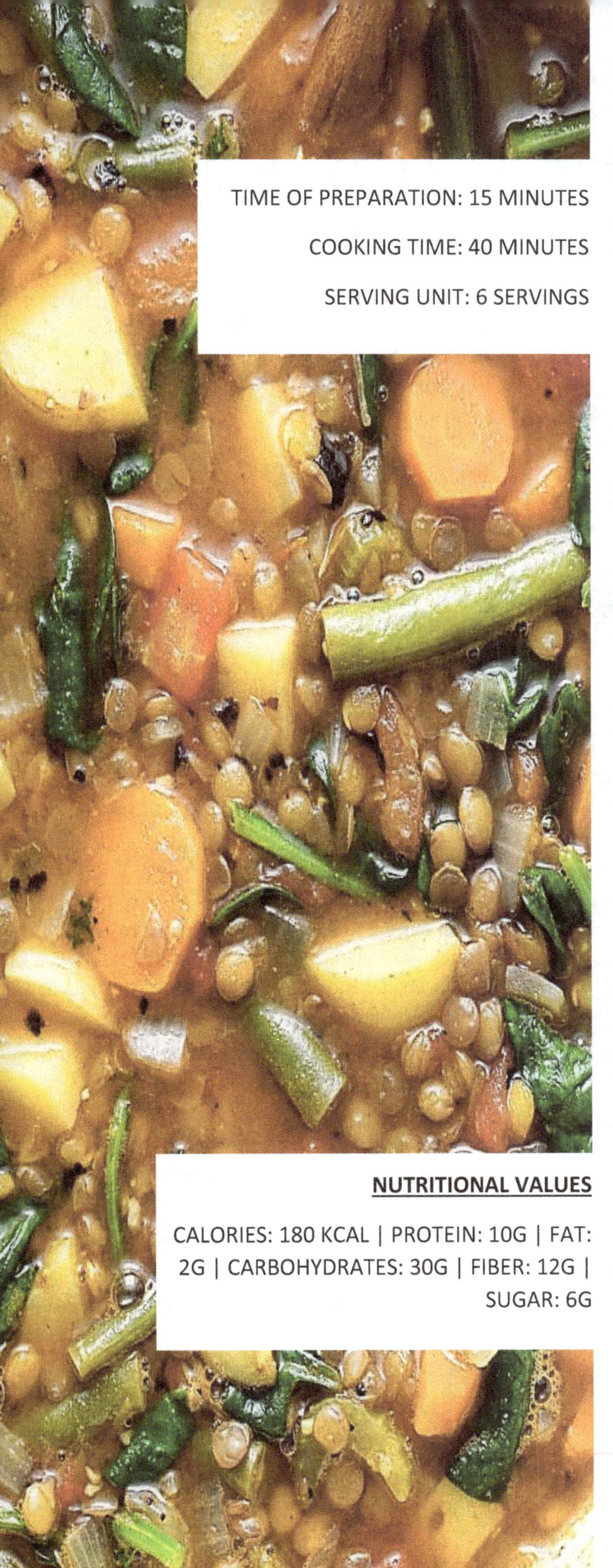

TIME OF PREPARATION: 15 MINUTES

COOKING TIME: 40 MINUTES

SERVING UNIT: 6 SERVINGS

**NUTRITIONAL VALUES**

CALORIES: 180 KCAL | PROTEIN: 10G | FAT: 2G | CARBOHYDRATES: 30G | FIBER: 12G | SUGAR: 6G

# LENTIL AND VEGETABLE SOUP

- 1 cup lentils, rinsed
- 1 onion, diced
- 2 carrots, diced
- 2 celery stalks, diced
- 2 cloves garlic, minced
- 1 can (14.5 oz) diced tomatoes
- 6 cups vegetable broth
- 1 teaspoon dried thyme
- 1 teaspoon cumin
- 1 bay leaf
- Salt and pepper to taste
- 2 cups spinach, chopped

## PROCEDURES

1. Sauté onion, carrots, and celery until softened.
2. Add garlic and cook for 1 minute.
3. Stir in lentils, tomatoes, broth, thyme, cumin, bay leaf, salt, and pepper.
4. Bring to a boil, reduce heat, and simmer for 30-35 minutes until lentils are tender.
5. Add spinach and cook for 5 minutes.
6. Remove bay leaf and serve.

## HEALTH BENEFITS

1. High in fiber: Promotes digestive health and satiety.
2. Plant-based protein: Lentils provide essential amino acids.
3. Low in fat: Supports heart health.

# HEARTY CHICKEN AND BARLEY STEW

TIME OF PREPARATION: 20 MINUTES

COOKING TIME: 1 HOUR

SERVING UNIT: 6 SERVINGS

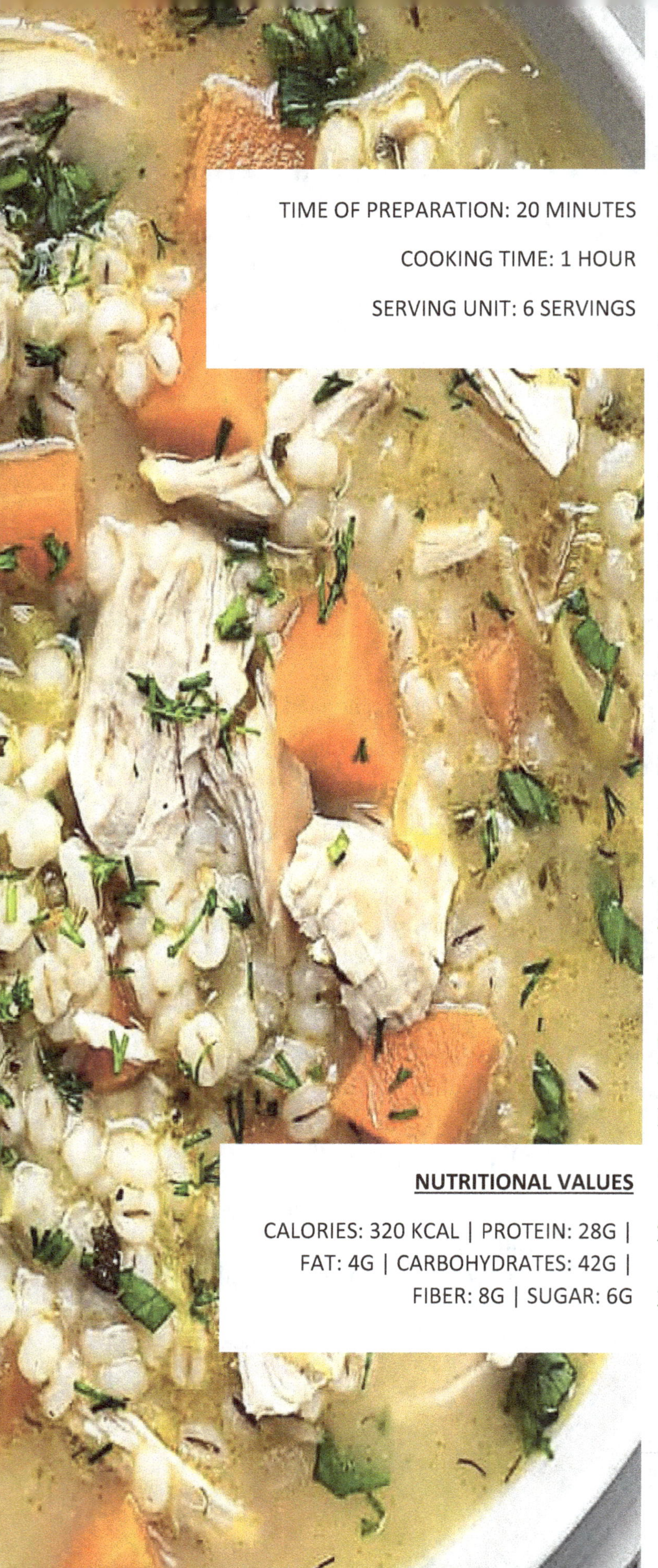

- 1 lb boneless, skinless chicken breasts, cubed
- 1 cup pearl barley
- 1 onion, diced
- 3 carrots, diced
- 2 celery stalks, diced
- 2 cloves garlic, minced
- 1 can (14.5 oz) diced tomatoes
- 6 cups low-sodium chicken broth
- 1 teaspoon dried thyme
- 1 teaspoon dried rosemary
- 1 bay leaf
- Salt and pepper to taste
- 2 cups kale, chopped

## PROCEDURES

1. Sauté chicken until browned, then set aside.
2. In the same pot, sauté onion, carrots, and celery until softened.
3. Add garlic and cook for 1 minute.
4. Stir in barley, tomatoes, broth, thyme, rosemary, bay leaf, salt, and pepper.
5. Return chicken to the pot, bring to a boil, then reduce heat and simmer for 45 minutes.
6. Add kale and cook for 5 more minutes.
7. Remove bay leaf and serve.

## HEALTH BENEFITS

1. High in protein: Supports muscle repair and growth.
2. Rich in fiber: Promotes digestive health and keeps you full longer.
3. Low in fat: Supports heart health.

### NUTRITIONAL VALUES

CALORIES: 320 KCAL | PROTEIN: 28G | FAT: 4G | CARBOHYDRATES: 42G | FIBER: 8G | SUGAR: 6G

# TOMATO BASIL SOUP

TIME OF PREPARATION: 10 MINUTES

COOKING TIME: 30 MINUTES

SERVING UNIT: 4 SERVINGS

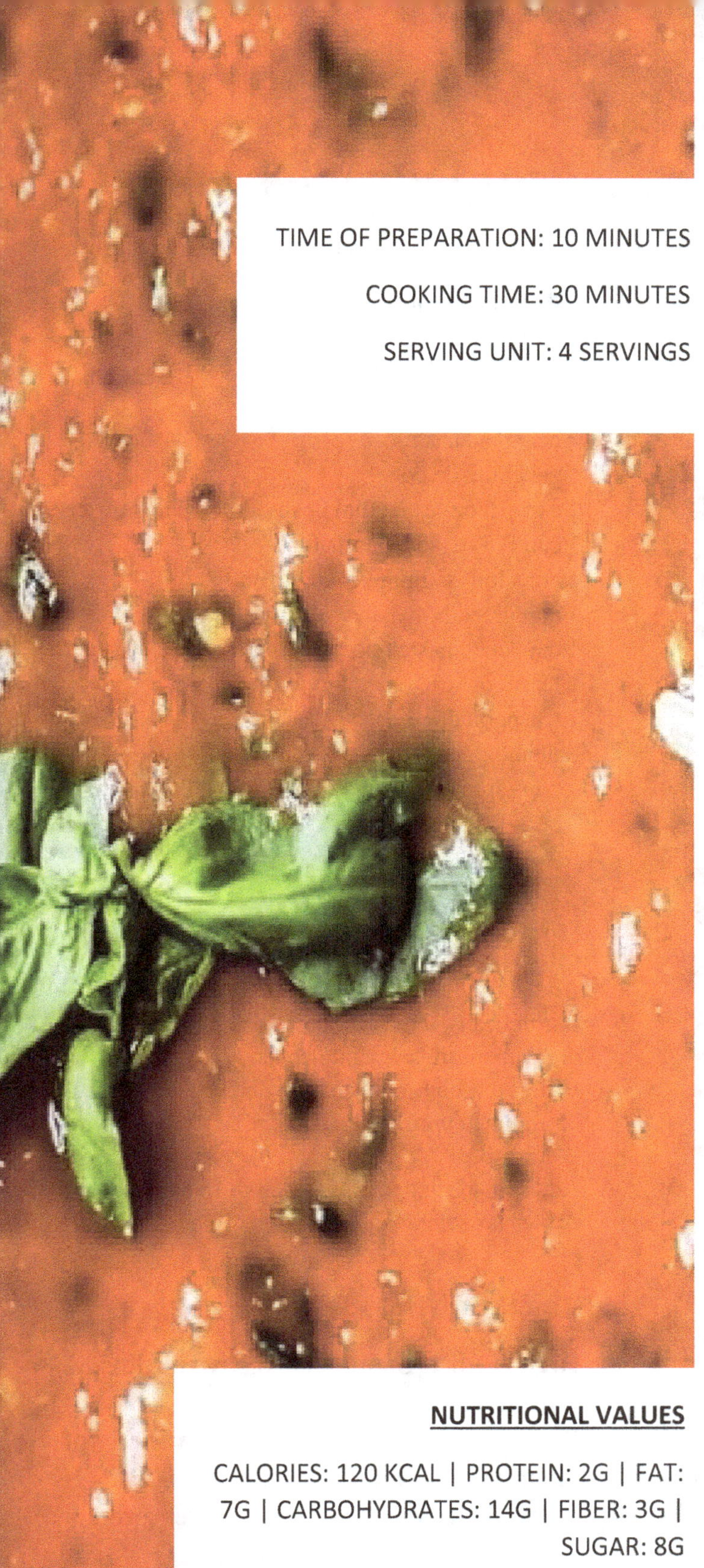

- 2 tablespoons olive oil
- 1 onion, chopped
- 2 cloves garlic, minced
- 1 can (28 oz) crushed tomatoes
- 2 cups low-sodium vegetable broth
- 1/2 cup fresh basil leaves, chopped
- 1 teaspoon dried oregano
- 1 teaspoon sugar (optional)
- Salt and pepper to taste

## PROCEDURES

1. Heat olive oil in a pot, sauté onion until translucent.
2. Add garlic and cook for 1 minute.
3. Stir in crushed tomatoes, broth, basil, oregano, sugar (if using), salt, and pepper.
4. Bring to a boil, reduce heat, and simmer for 20-25 minutes.
5. Blend the soup until smooth using an immersion blender.
6. Adjust seasoning if needed and serve.

## HEALTH BENEFITS

Low in calories: Supports weight management.

Rich in antioxidants: Tomatoes and basil provide lycopene and other beneficial compounds.

Heart-healthy fats: Olive oil contributes to cardiovascular health.

**NUTRITIONAL VALUES**

CALORIES: 120 KCAL | PROTEIN: 2G | FAT: 7G | CARBOHYDRATES: 14G | FIBER: 3G | SUGAR: 8G

# MINESTRONE SOUP

TIME OF PREPARATION: 15 MINUTES

COOKING TIME: 45 MINUTES

SERVING UNIT: 6 SERVINGS

- 2 tablespoons olive oil
- 1 onion, diced
- 2 cloves garlic, minced
- 2 carrots, diced
- 2 celery stalks, diced
- 1 zucchini, diced
- 1 can (15 oz) cannellini beans, drained and rinsed
- 1 can (15 oz) diced tomatoes
- 4 cups low-sodium vegetable broth
- 1 cup green beans, cut into 1-inch pieces
- 1 cup small pasta (e.g., ditalini)
- 1 teaspoon dried oregano
- 1 teaspoon dried basil
- Salt and pepper to taste
- 2 cups spinach, chopped

## PROCEDURES

1. Heat olive oil in a large pot, sauté onion, garlic, carrots, and celery until soft.
2. Add zucchini and cook for 5 minutes.
3. Stir in beans, tomatoes, broth, green beans, pasta, oregano, basil, salt, and pepper.
4. Bring to a boil, reduce heat, and simmer for 20-25 minutes until vegetables are tender and pasta is cooked.
5. Add spinach and cook for 5 more minutes.
6. Adjust seasoning and serve.

## HEALTH BENEFITS

1. High in fiber: Supports digestive health and satiety.
2. Rich in vitamins: Provides a variety of vitamins from multiple vegetables.
3. Plant-based protein: Beans offer protein without the saturated fat of meat.

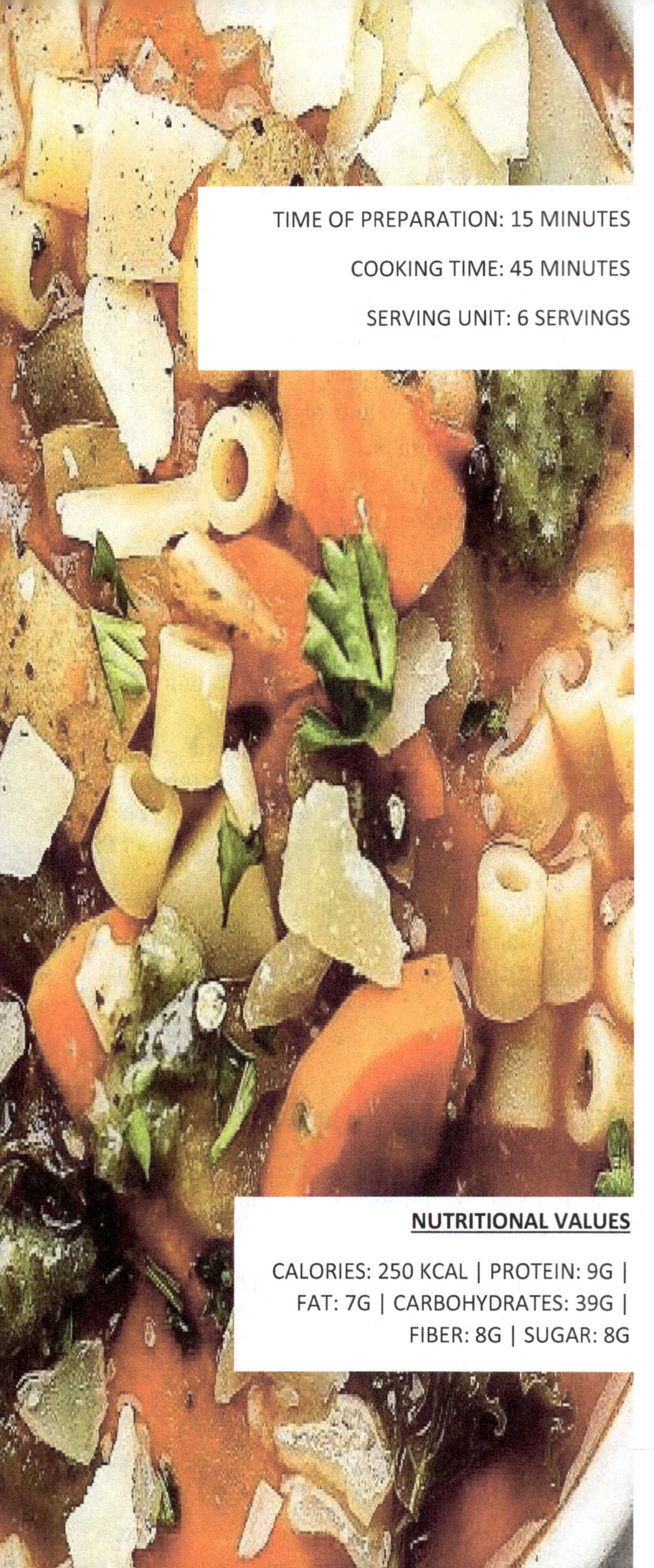

### NUTRITIONAL VALUES

CALORIES: 250 KCAL | PROTEIN: 9G | FAT: 7G | CARBOHYDRATES: 39G | FIBER: 8G | SUGAR: 8G

# SWEET POTATO AND BLACK BEAN CHILI

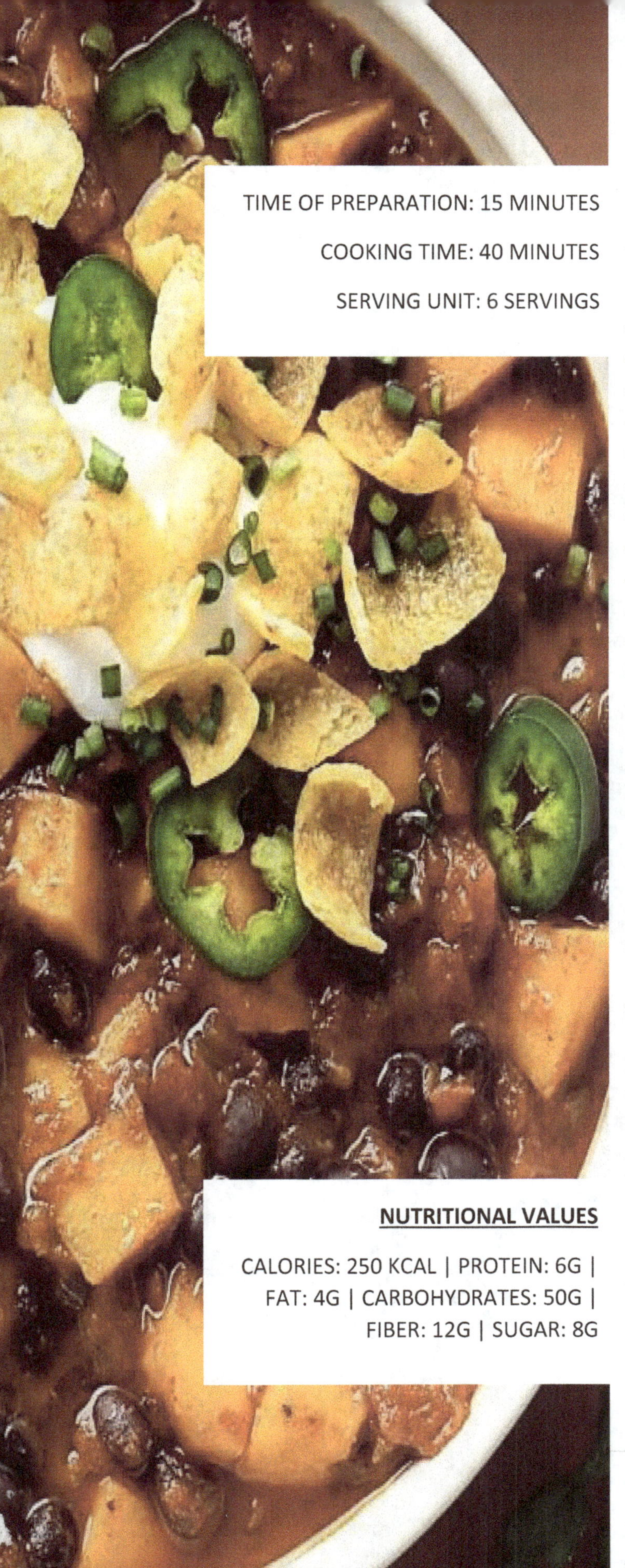

TIME OF PREPARATION: 15 MINUTES

COOKING TIME: 40 MINUTES

SERVING UNIT: 6 SERVINGS

- 1 tablespoon olive oil
- 1 onion, diced
- 2 cloves garlic, minced
- 1 bell pepper, diced
- 2 sweet potatoes, peeled and diced
- 1 can (15 oz) black beans, drained and rinsed
- 1 can (15 oz) diced tomatoes
- 2 cups low-sodium vegetable broth
- 1 teaspoon chili powder
- 1 teaspoon cumin
- 1/2 teaspoon paprika
- Salt and pepper to taste
- 1 cup corn kernels (fresh or frozen)
- 1/4 cup fresh cilantro, chopped

## PROCEDURES

1. Heat olive oil in a large pot, sauté onion, garlic, and bell pepper until softened.
2. Add sweet potatoes and cook for 5 minutes.
3. Stir in black beans, tomatoes, broth, chili powder, cumin, paprika, salt, and pepper.
4. Bring to a boil, reduce heat, and simmer for 25-30 minutes until sweet potatoes are tender.
5. Add corn and cook for another 5 minutes.
6. Stir in cilantro before serving.

## HEALTH BENEFITS

1. High in fiber: Promotes digestive health and satiety.
2. Rich in vitamins: Sweet potatoes provide vitamin A and C.
3. Plant-based protein: Black beans offer protein and essential nutrients.

### NUTRITIONAL VALUES

CALORIES: 250 KCAL | PROTEIN: 6G | FAT: 4G | CARBOHYDRATES: 50G | FIBER: 12G | SUGAR: 8G

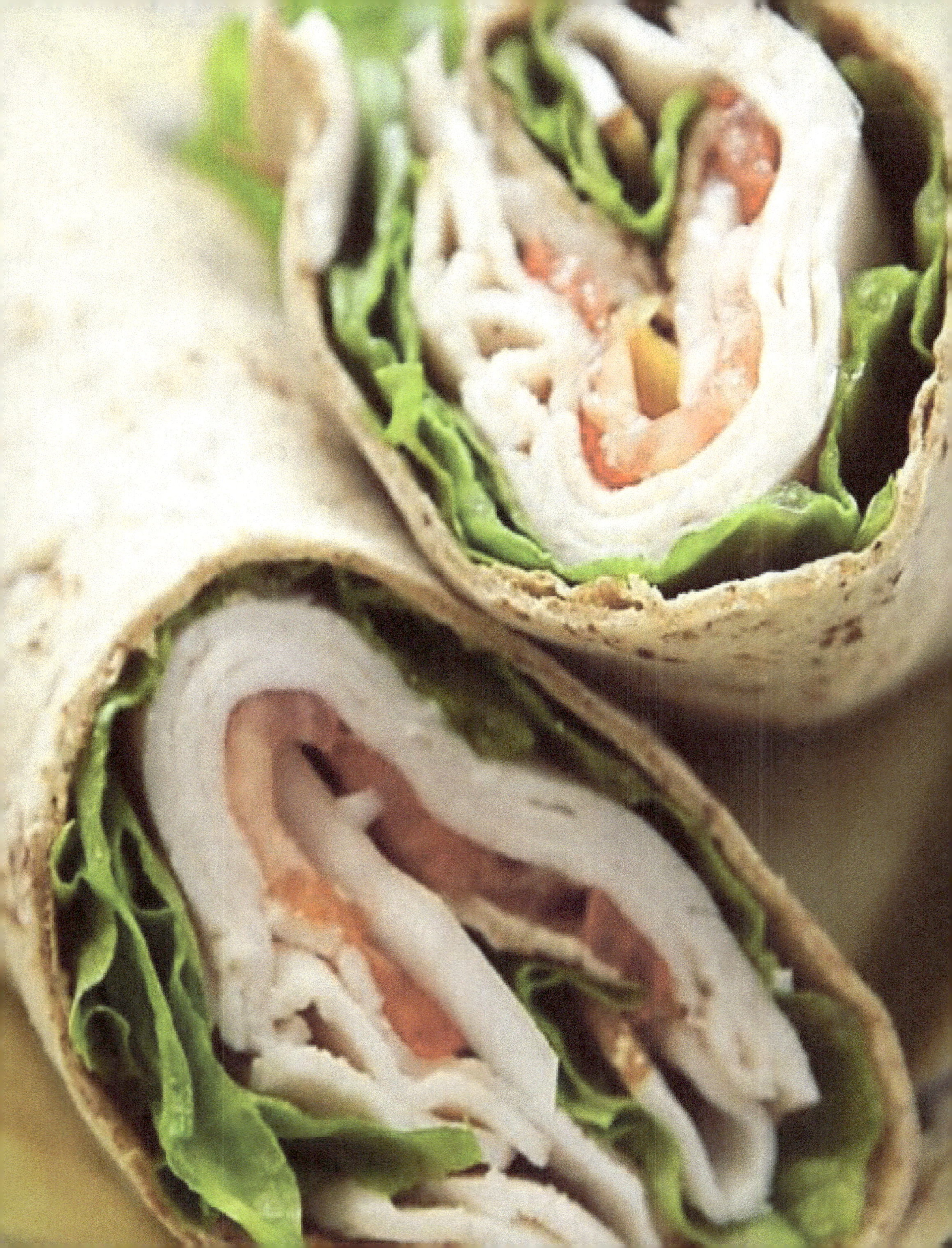

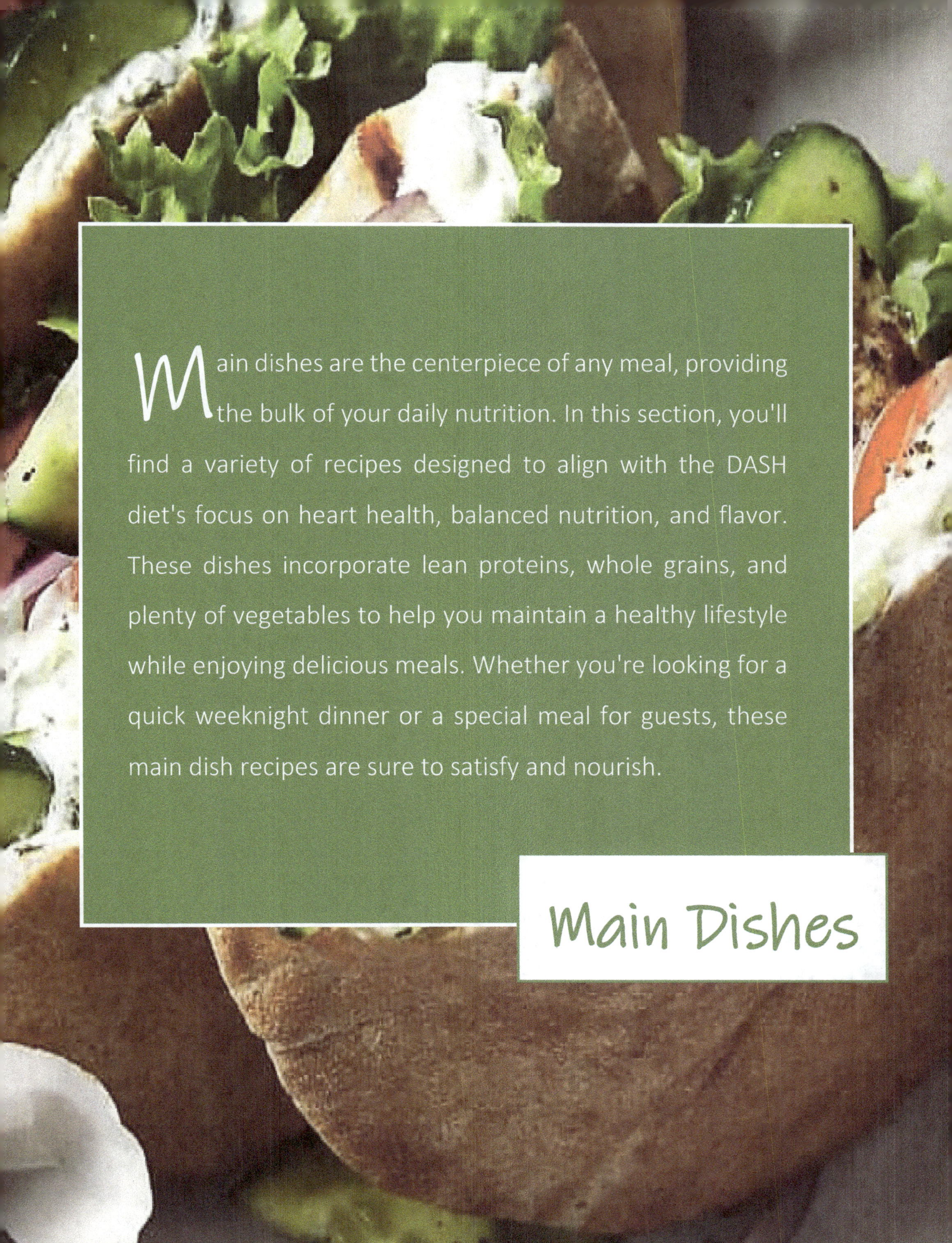

Main dishes are the centerpiece of any meal, providing the bulk of your daily nutrition. In this section, you'll find a variety of recipes designed to align with the DASH diet's focus on heart health, balanced nutrition, and flavor. These dishes incorporate lean proteins, whole grains, and plenty of vegetables to help you maintain a healthy lifestyle while enjoying delicious meals. Whether you're looking for a quick weeknight dinner or a special meal for guests, these main dish recipes are sure to satisfy and nourish.

# Main Dishes

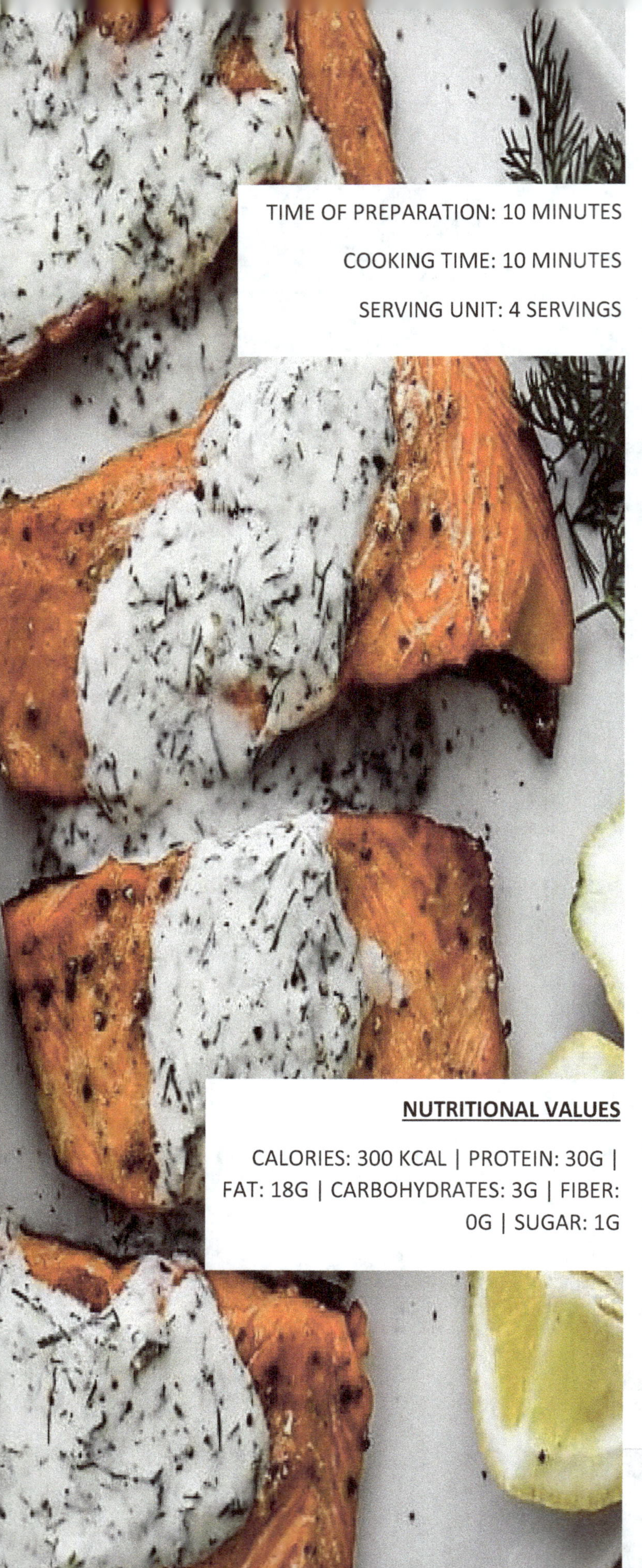

TIME OF PREPARATION: 10 MINUTES

COOKING TIME: 10 MINUTES

SERVING UNIT: 4 SERVINGS

**NUTRITIONAL VALUES**

CALORIES: 300 KCAL | PROTEIN: 30G |
FAT: 18G | CARBOHYDRATES: 3G | FIBER:
0G | SUGAR: 1G

# GRILLED SALMON WITH LEMON-DILL SAUCE

- 4 salmon fillets
- Olive oil
- Salt and pepper
- 1/4 cup plain Greek yogurt
- Juice and zest of 1 lemon
- 1 tablespoon fresh dill, chopped
- 1 garlic clove, minced

## PROCEDURES

1. Preheat grill to medium-high heat.
2. Brush salmon fillets with olive oil and season with salt and pepper.
3. Grill salmon for 4-5 minutes per side, or until cooked through.
4. In a bowl, mix Greek yogurt, lemon juice and zest, dill, and garlic.
5. Serve grilled salmon with lemon-dill sauce on the side.

## HEALTH BENEFITS

1. Rich in omega-3 fatty acids: Supports heart and brain health.
2. High in protein: Helps with muscle repair and growth.
3. Low in carbohydrates: Suitable for maintaining balanced blood sugar levels.

# QUINOA-STUFFED BELL PEPPERS

TIME OF PREPARATION: 20 MINUTES

COOKING TIME: 40 MINUTES

SERVING UNIT: 4 SERVINGS

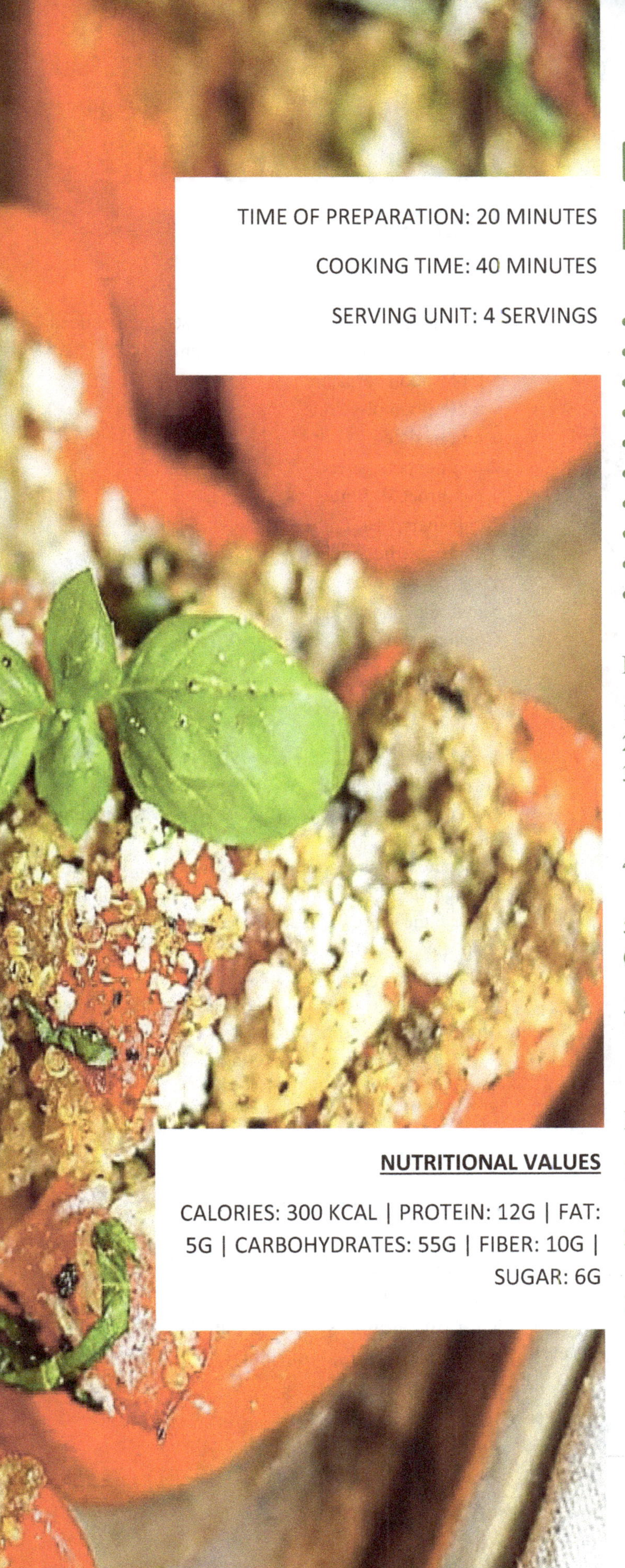

- 4 bell peppers, tops cut off and seeds removed
- 1 cup quinoa, rinsed
- 1 can (15 oz) black beans, drained and rinsed
- 1 cup corn kernels (fresh or frozen)
- 1/2 cup diced tomatoes
- 1/2 teaspoon cumin
- 1/2 teaspoon chili powder
- Salt and pepper to taste
- 1/4 cup shredded cheddar cheese (optional)
- Fresh cilantro, chopped (for garnish)

## PROCEDURES

1. Preheat oven to 375°F (190°C).
2. Cook quinoa according to package instructions.
3. In a large bowl, mix cooked quinoa, black beans, corn, diced tomatoes, cumin, chili powder, salt, and pepper.
4. Stuff bell peppers with quinoa mixture and place in a baking dish.
5. Cover with foil and bake for 30 minutes.
6. Remove foil, sprinkle with cheese if desired, and bake uncovered for an additional 10 minutes.
7. Garnish with fresh cilantro before serving.

## HEALTH BENEFITS

1. High in fiber: Promotes digestive health and keeps you full longer.
2. Plant-based protein: Quinoa and black beans provide essential amino acids.
3. Low in fat: Suitable for heart health and weight management.

### NUTRITIONAL VALUES

CALORIES: 300 KCAL | PROTEIN: 12G | FAT: 5G | CARBOHYDRATES: 55G | FIBER: 10G | SUGAR: 6G

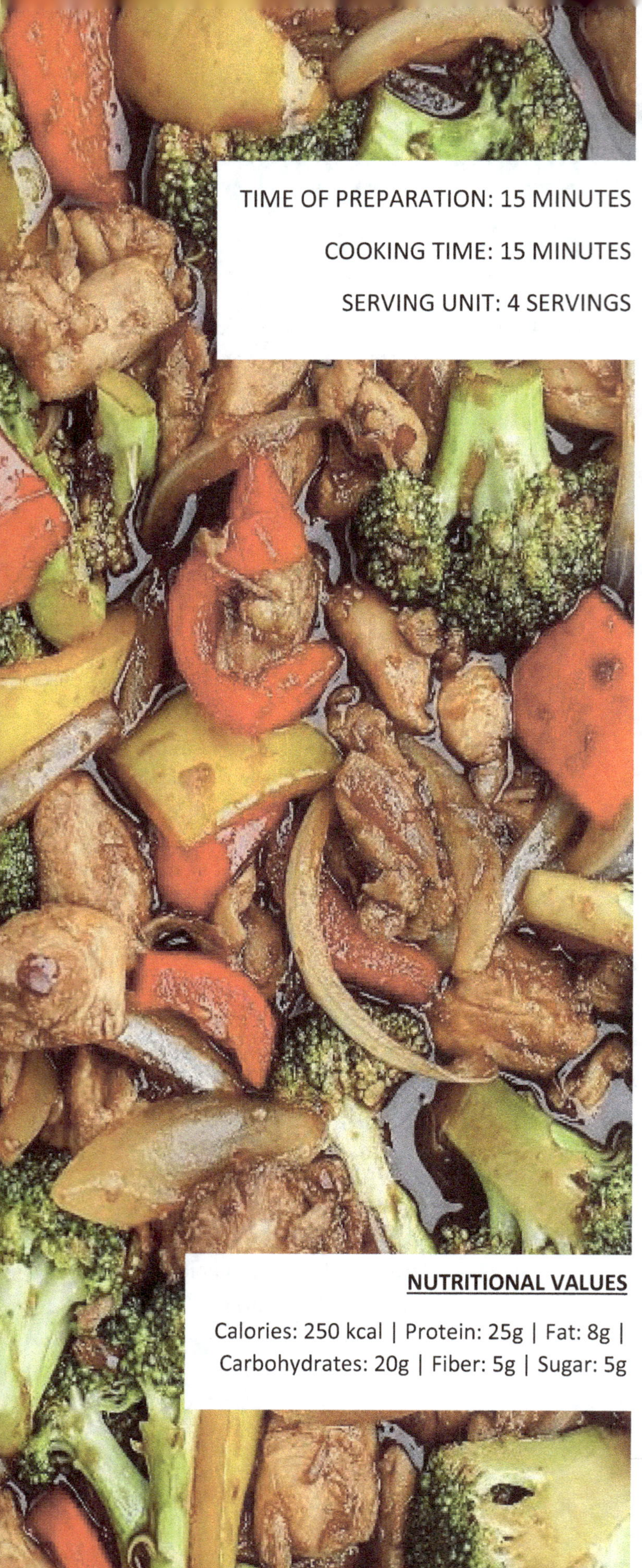

TIME OF PREPARATION: 15 MINUTES

COOKING TIME: 15 MINUTES

SERVING UNIT: 4 SERVINGS

**NUTRITIONAL VALUES**

Calories: 250 kcal | Protein: 25g | Fat: 8g | Carbohydrates: 20g | Fiber: 5g | Sugar: 5g

# CHICKEN AND VEGETABLE STIR-FRY

- 1 lb boneless, skinless chicken breasts, thinly sliced
- 2 tablespoons soy sauce (low-sodium)
- 1 tablespoon cornstarch
- 1 tablespoon olive oil
- 1 onion, sliced
- 2 bell peppers, sliced
- 1 cup broccoli florets
- 1 cup snap peas
- 2 cloves garlic, minced
- 1 teaspoon grated ginger
- Salt and pepper to taste
- Cooked brown rice or quinoa (optional, for serving)

## PROCEDURES

1. In a bowl, mix chicken with soy sauce and cornstarch, set aside.
2. Heat olive oil in a large skillet or wok over medium-high heat.
3. Add chicken and cook until browned and cooked through, about 5-7 minutes. Remove from skillet.
4. In the same skillet, add onion, bell peppers, broccoli, snap peas, garlic, and ginger. Stir-fry for 5-7 minutes until vegetables are tender-crisp.
5. Return chicken to the skillet, season with salt and pepper, and toss to combine.
6. Serve immediately over cooked brown rice or quinoa if desired.

## HEALTH BENEFITS

1. High in protein: Supports muscle repair and growth.
2. Low in fat: Suitable for heart health and weight management.
3. Rich in vitamins and minerals: Vegetables provide essential nutrients like vitamin C, potassium, and fiber.

# BAKED COD WITH HERB CRUST

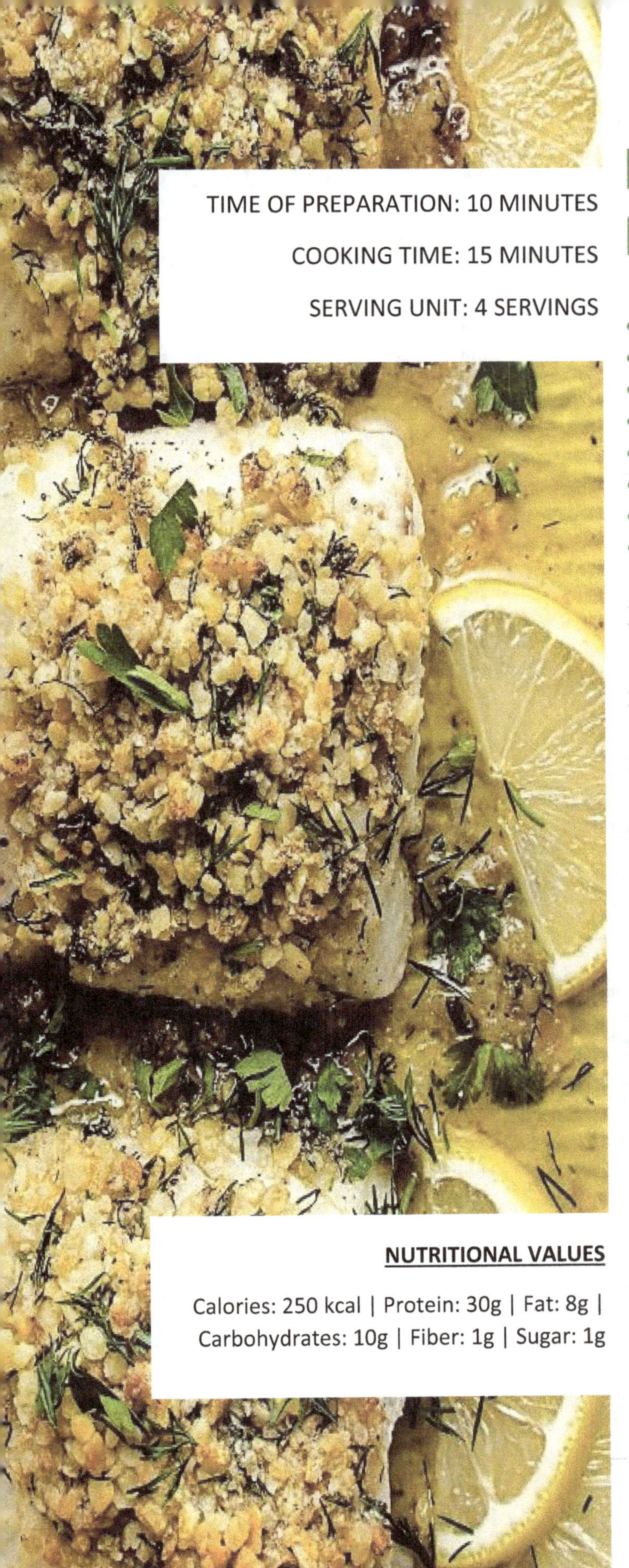

TIME OF PREPARATION: 10 MINUTES

COOKING TIME: 15 MINUTES

SERVING UNIT: 4 SERVINGS

- 4 cod fillets (about 6 oz each)
- 1/4 cup whole wheat breadcrumbs
- 2 tablespoons chopped fresh parsley
- 1 tablespoon chopped fresh dill
- 1 tablespoon olive oil
- 1 tablespoon Dijon mustard
- Salt and pepper to taste
- Lemon wedges (for serving)

## PROCEDURES

1. Preheat oven to 400°F (200°C).
2. In a bowl, combine breadcrumbs, parsley, dill, olive oil, and mustard.
3. Pat dry cod fillets and season with salt and pepper.
4. Place cod fillets on a baking sheet lined with parchment paper.
5. Spread herb mixture evenly over the top of each fillet, pressing lightly to adhere.
6. Bake for 12-15 minutes, or until fish flakes easily with a fork.
7. Serve hot with lemon wedges.

## HEALTH BENEFITS

1. High in protein: Supports muscle repair and growth.
2. Low in fat: Suitable for heart health and weight management.
3. Rich in omega-3 fatty acids: Promotes heart and brain health.

### NUTRITIONAL VALUES

Calories: 250 kcal | Protein: 30g | Fat: 8g | Carbohydrates: 10g | Fiber: 1g | Sugar: 1g

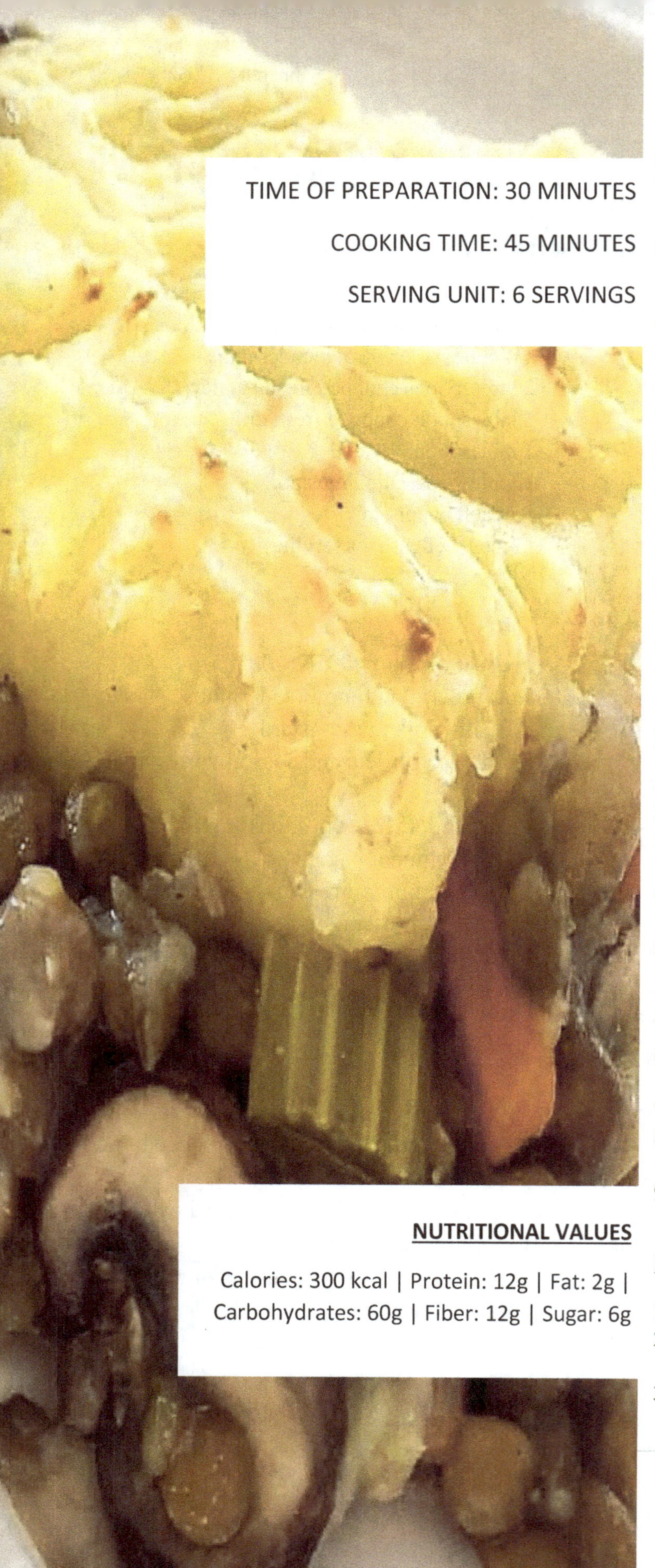

TIME OF PREPARATION: 30 MINUTES

COOKING TIME: 45 MINUTES

SERVING UNIT: 6 SERVINGS

**NUTRITIONAL VALUES**

Calories: 300 kcal | Protein: 12g | Fat: 2g |
Carbohydrates: 60g | Fiber: 12g | Sugar: 6g

# LENTIL AND MUSHROOM SHEPHERD'S PIE

- 2 cups cooked lentils
- 1 onion, diced
- 2 cloves garlic, minced
- 2 carrots, diced
- 2 celery stalks, diced
- 8 oz mushrooms, sliced
- 1 cup frozen peas
- 1 tablespoon tomato paste
- 1 tablespoon Worcestershire sauce (optional)
- 1 teaspoon dried thyme
- Salt and pepper to taste
- 4 cups mashed potatoes (prepared)
- Fresh parsley, chopped (for garnish)

## PROCEDURES

1. Preheat oven to 375°F (190°C).
2. Heat olive oil in a large skillet over medium heat.
3. Sauté onion, garlic, carrots, and celery until softened, about 5-7 minutes.
4. Add mushrooms and cook until they release their moisture, about 5 minutes.
5. Stir in cooked lentils, frozen peas, tomato paste, Worcestershire sauce (if using), thyme, salt, and pepper. Cook for another 5 minutes, stirring occasionally.
6. Transfer lentil and mushroom mixture to a baking dish.
7. Spread mashed potatoes evenly over the top.
8. Bake for 25-30 minutes, or until heated through and lightly browned on top.
9. Garnish with fresh parsley before serving.

## HEALTH BENEFITS

1. High in fiber: Promotes digestive health and satiety.
2. Plant-based protein: Lentils provide essential amino acids.
3. Low in fat: Suitable for heart health and weight management.

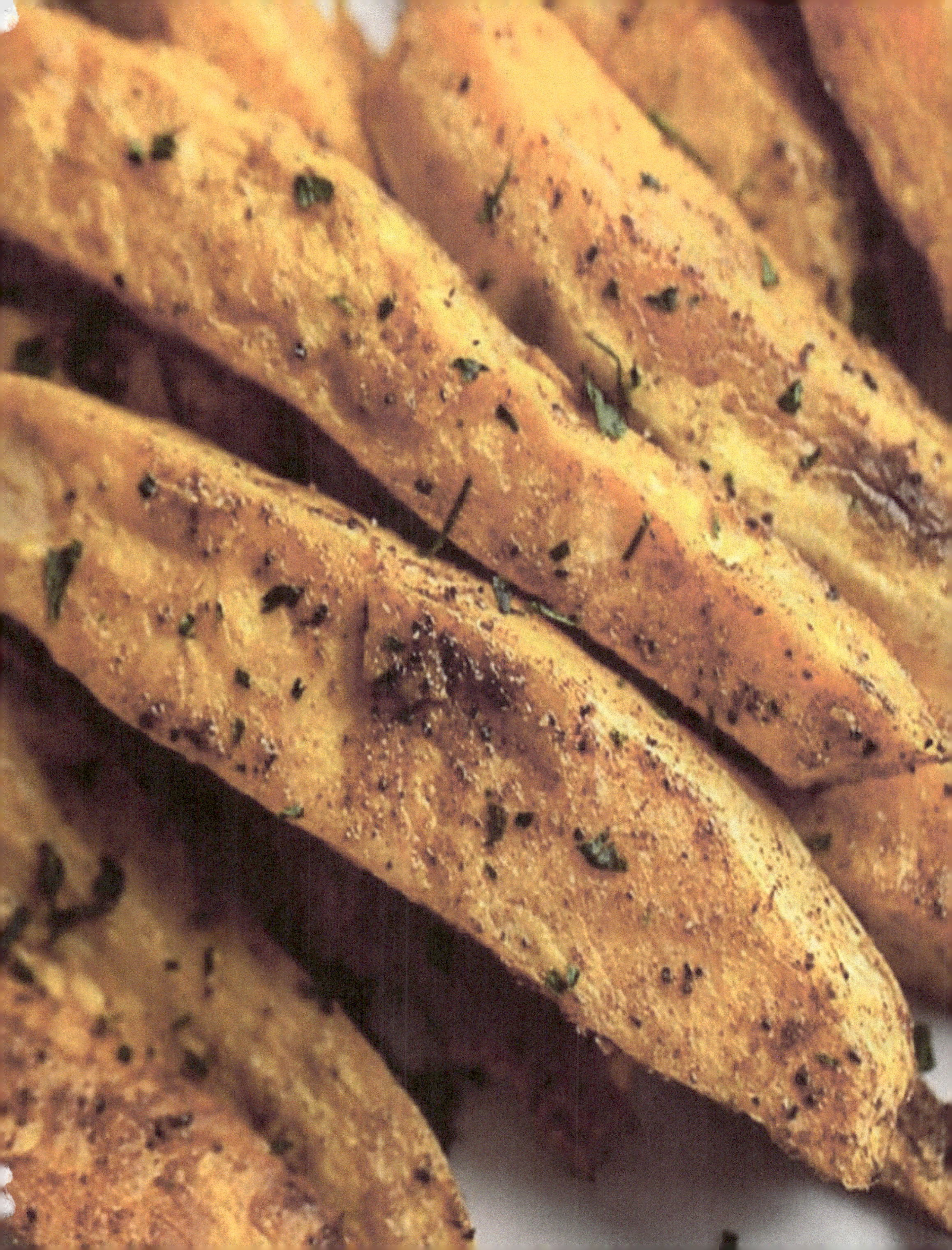

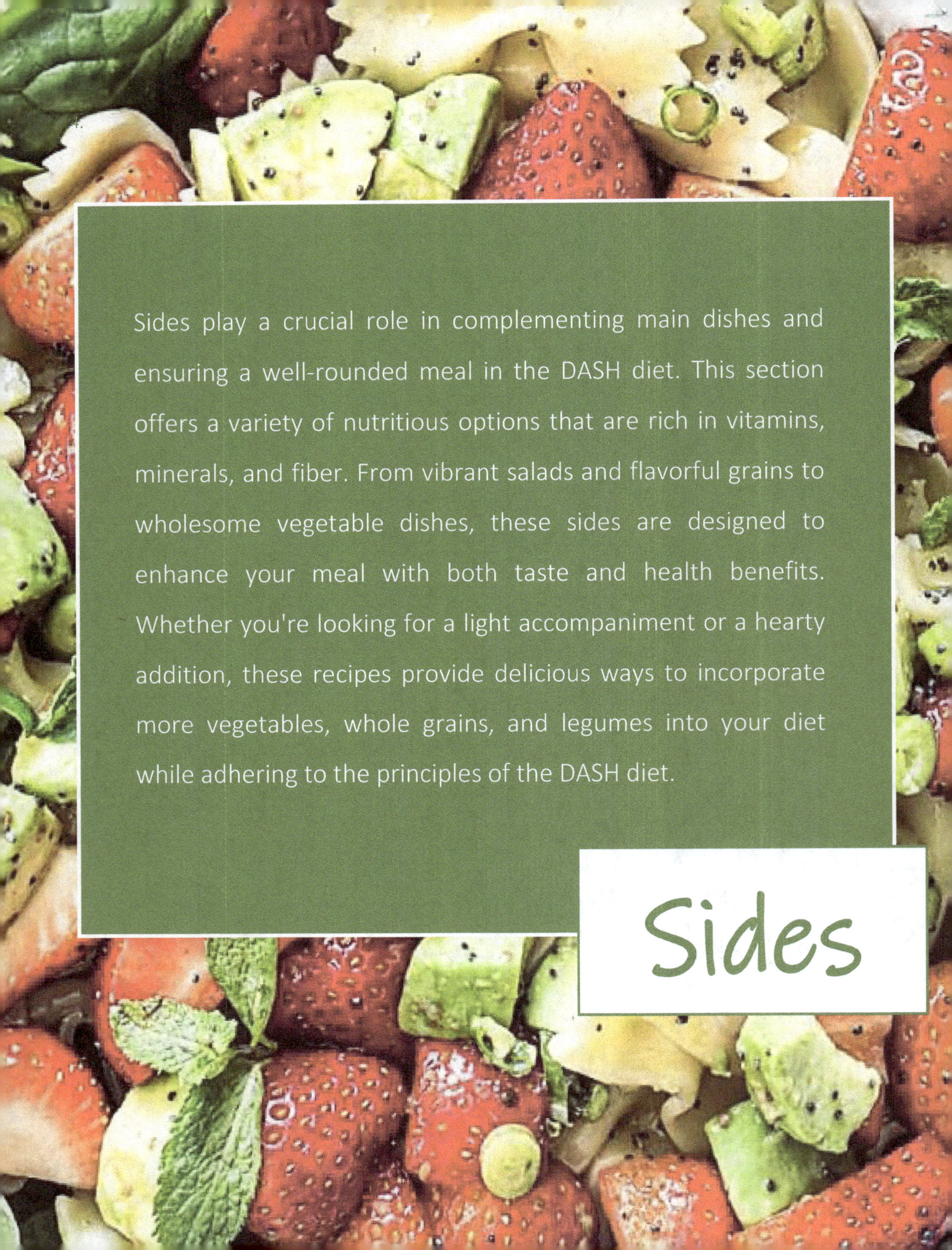

Sides play a crucial role in complementing main dishes and ensuring a well-rounded meal in the DASH diet. This section offers a variety of nutritious options that are rich in vitamins, minerals, and fiber. From vibrant salads and flavorful grains to wholesome vegetable dishes, these sides are designed to enhance your meal with both taste and health benefits. Whether you're looking for a light accompaniment or a hearty addition, these recipes provide delicious ways to incorporate more vegetables, whole grains, and legumes into your diet while adhering to the principles of the DASH diet.

# Sides

# GARLIC AND HERB ROASTED VEGETABLES

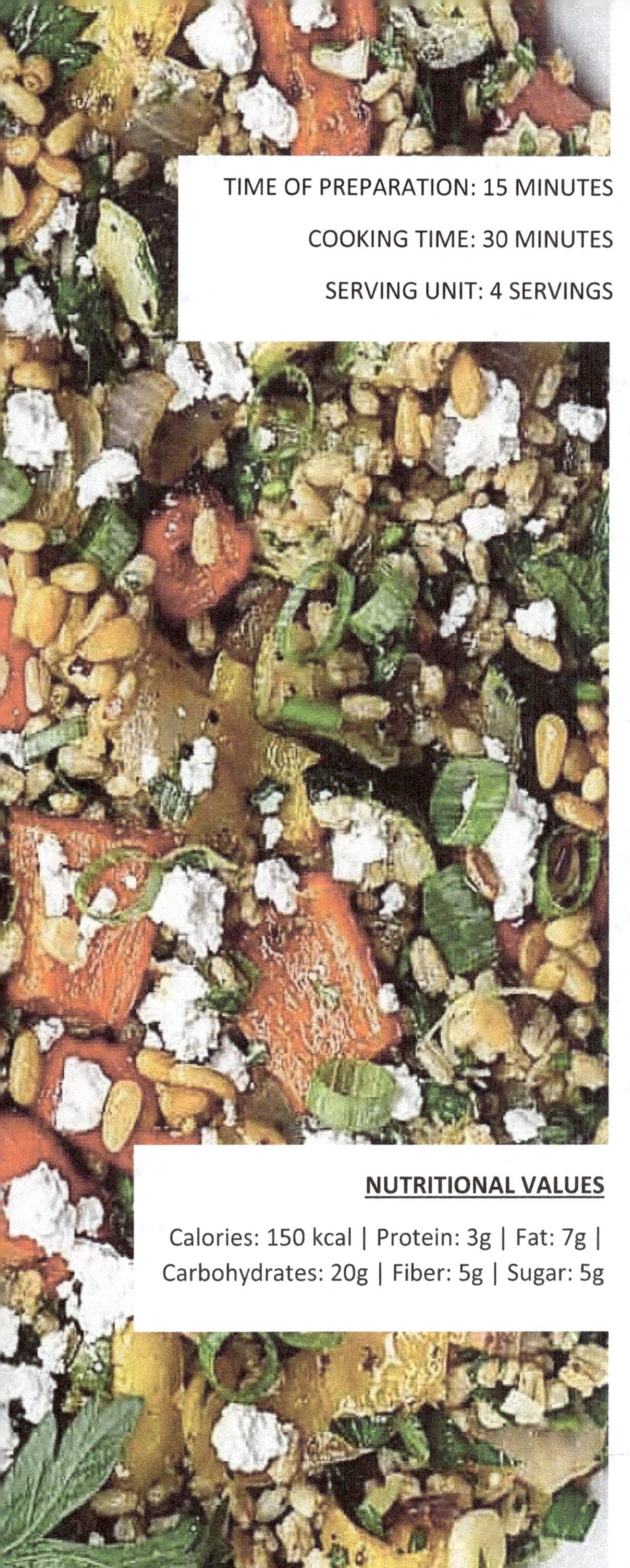

TIME OF PREPARATION: 15 MINUTES

COOKING TIME: 30 MINUTES

SERVING UNIT: 4 SERVINGS

- 1 lb mixed vegetables (such as carrots, bell peppers, zucchini, and broccoli), cut into bite-sized pieces
- 2 tablespoons olive oil
- 4 cloves garlic, minced
- 1 teaspoon dried thyme
- 1 teaspoon dried rosemary
- Salt and pepper to taste

## PROCEDURES

1. Preheat oven to 400°F (200°C).
2. In a large bowl, toss mixed vegetables with olive oil, garlic, thyme, rosemary, salt, and pepper until evenly coated.
3. Spread vegetables in a single layer on a baking sheet lined with parchment paper.
4. Roast in the oven for 25-30 minutes, stirring halfway through, until vegetables are tender and lightly browned.

## HEALTH BENEFITS

1. High in fiber: Promotes digestive health and helps with satiety.
2. Rich in vitamins and minerals: Provides essential nutrients like vitamin C, vitamin A, and potassium.
3. Olive oil contributes to a balanced diet.

### NUTRITIONAL VALUES

Calories: 150 kcal | Protein: 3g | Fat: 7g | Carbohydrates: 20g | Fiber: 5g | Sugar: 5g

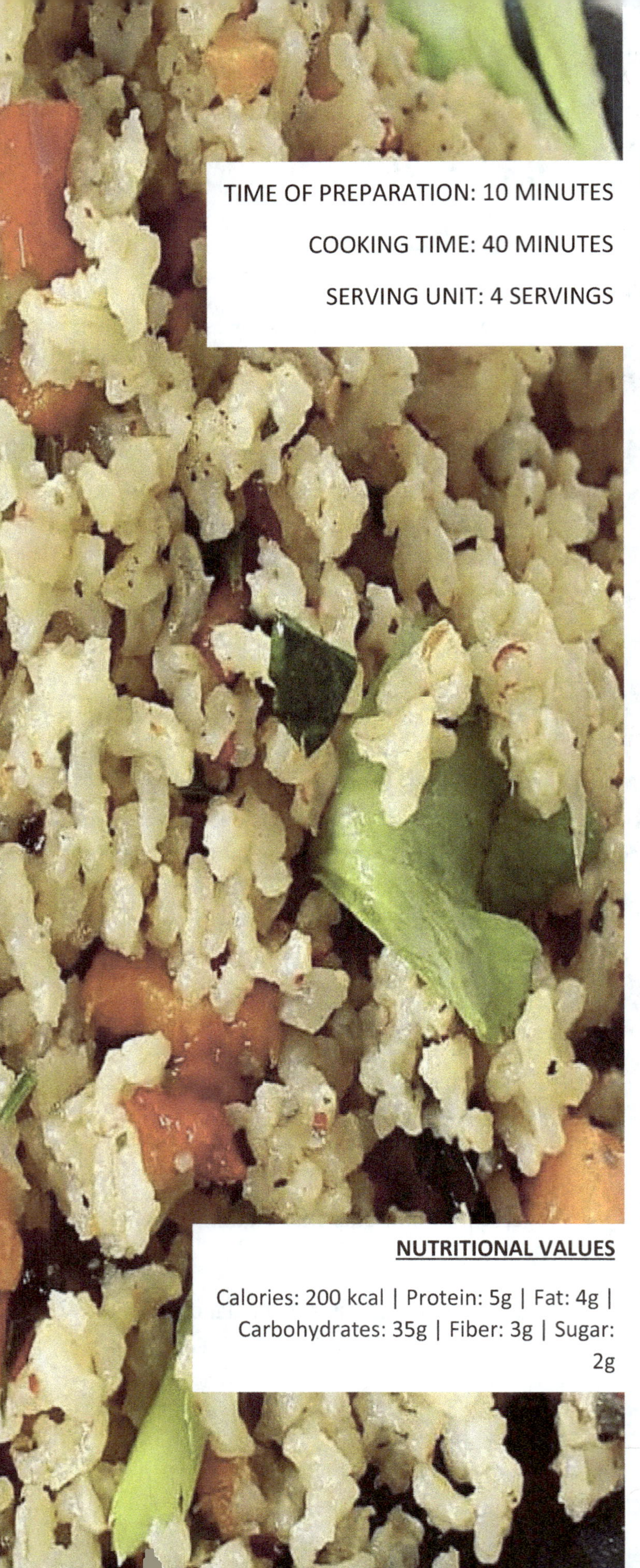

TIME OF PREPARATION: 10 MINUTES

COOKING TIME: 40 MINUTES

SERVING UNIT: 4 SERVINGS

**NUTRITIONAL VALUES**

Calories: 200 kcal | Protein: 5g | Fat: 4g | Carbohydrates: 35g | Fiber: 3g | Sugar: 2g

# BROWN RICE PILAF

- 1 cup brown rice
- 2 cups low-sodium chicken or vegetable broth
- 1 tablespoon olive oil
- 1 onion, finely chopped
- 2 cloves garlic, minced
- 1 carrot, diced
- 1 celery stalk, diced
- 1/4 cup chopped parsley (optional)
- Salt and pepper to taste

## PROCEDURES

1. Rinse brown rice under cold water until water runs clear.
2. In a saucepan, heat olive oil over medium heat. Add onion and garlic, sauté until softened.
3. Add brown rice, stirring constantly for 2 minutes.
4. Add broth, bring to a boil, then reduce heat to low. Cover and simmer for 35-40 minutes, or until rice is tender and liquid is absorbed.
5. Stir in carrot, celery, and parsley (if using). Season with salt and pepper to taste.
6. Remove from heat, let sit covered for 5 minutes before serving.

## HEALTH BENEFITS

1. High in fiber: Supports digestive health and helps with satiety.
2. Low in fat: Suitable for heart health and weight management.
3. Provides essential vitamins and minerals: Brown rice is rich in manganese, selenium, and magnesium.

# STEAMED ASPARAGUS WITH LEMON ZEST

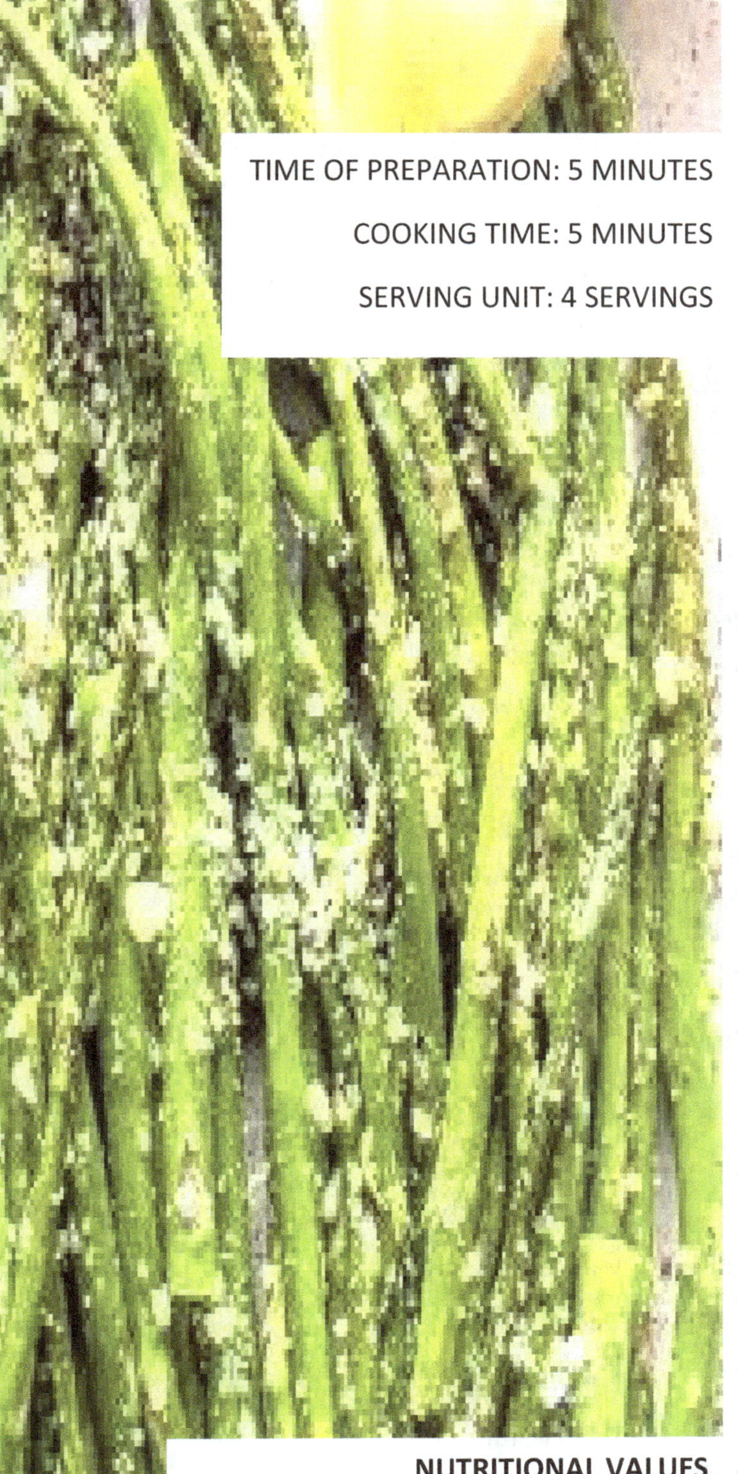

TIME OF PREPARATION: 5 MINUTES

COOKING TIME: 5 MINUTES

SERVING UNIT: 4 SERVINGS

- 1 lb asparagus, ends trimmed
- Zest of 1 lemon
- Salt and pepper to taste

## PROCEDURES

1. Fill a large pot with 1-2 inches of water and place a steamer basket inside.
2. Bring water to a boil over medium-high heat.
3. Add asparagus to the steamer basket, cover, and steam for 4-5 minutes, or until asparagus is tender-crisp.
4. Remove asparagus from steamer basket and transfer to a serving dish.
5. Sprinkle with lemon zest, salt, and pepper.

## HEALTH BENEFITS

1. Low in calories: Suitable for weight management and overall health.
2. High in fiber: Promotes digestive health and helps with satiety.
3. Rich in vitamins and minerals: Asparagus is a good source of folate, vitamin K, and antioxidants.

### NUTRITIONAL VALUES

Calories: 25 kcal | Protein: 2g | Fat: 0g | Carbohydrates: 5g | Fiber: 3g | Sugar: 2g

# SWEET POTATO WEDGES

TIME OF PREPARATION: 10 MINUTES

COOKING TIME: 30 MINUTES

SERVING UNIT: 4 SERVINGS

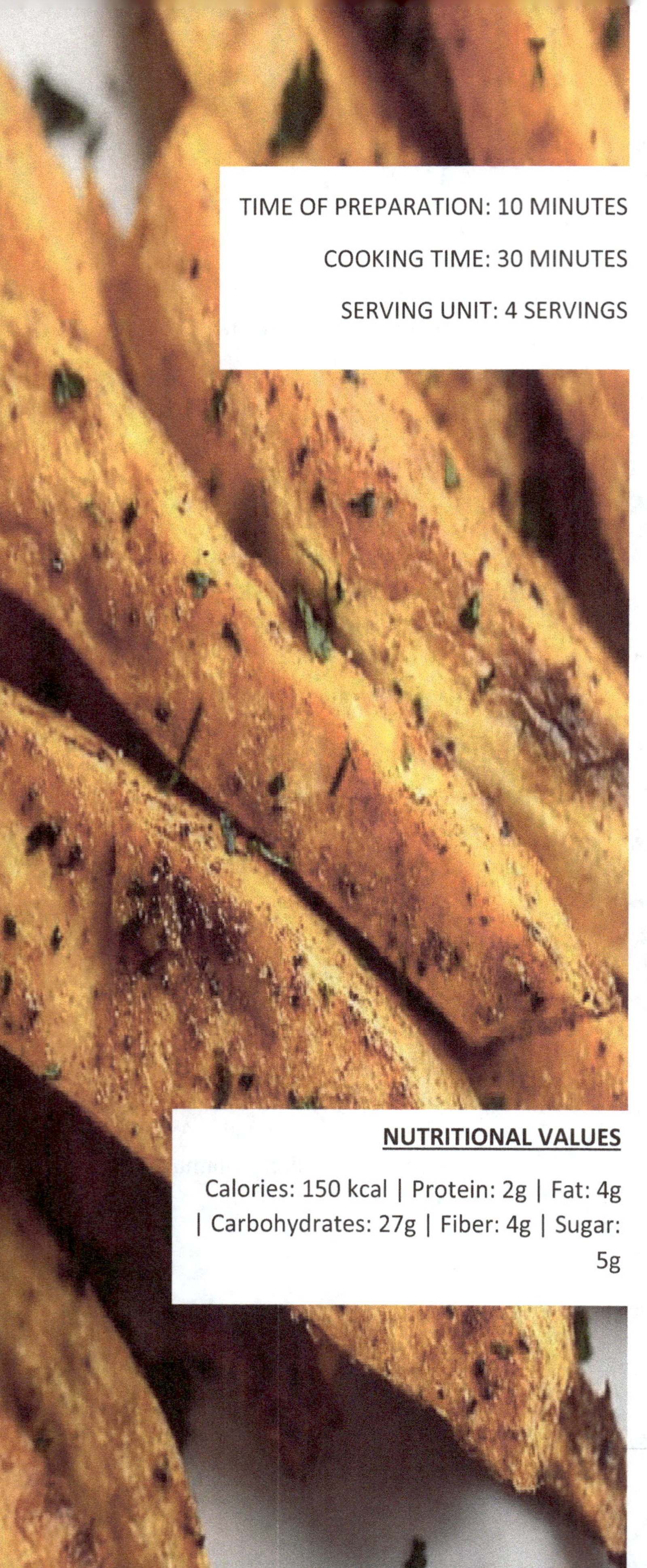

- 2 large sweet potatoes, washed and cut into wedges
- 1 tablespoon olive oil
- 1 teaspoon paprika
- 1/2 teaspoon garlic powder
- Salt and pepper to taste

## PROCEDURES

1. Preheat oven to 400°F (200°C).
2. In a large bowl, toss sweet potato wedges with olive oil, paprika, garlic powder, salt, and pepper until evenly coated.
3. Spread wedges in a single layer on a baking sheet lined with parchment paper.
4. Bake for 25-30 minutes, flipping halfway through, until wedges are tender and crispy.

## HEALTH BENEFITS

1. High in fiber: Promotes digestive health and helps with satiety.
2. Rich in vitamins and minerals: Sweet potatoes provide vitamin A, vitamin C, and potassium.
3. Low glycemic index: Helps regulate blood sugar levels.

## NUTRITIONAL VALUES

Calories: 150 kcal | Protein: 2g | Fat: 4g | Carbohydrates: 27g | Fiber: 4g | Sugar: 5g

# MIXED GREEN BEANS WITH ALMONDS

TIME OF PREPARATION: 10 MINUTES

COOKING TIME: 10 MINUTES

SERVING UNIT: 4 SERVINGS

- 1 lb green beans, trimmed
- 1/4 cup sliced almonds
- 1 tablespoon olive oil
- 2 cloves garlic, minced
- Salt and pepper to taste

## PROCEDURES

1. Bring a large pot of water to a boil.
2. Add green beans and cook for 3-4 minutes, until tender-crisp. Drain and set aside.
3. In a large skillet, heat olive oil over medium heat.
4. Add minced garlic and sauté for 1 minute until fragrant.
5. Add cooked green beans and sliced almonds to the skillet. Stir-fry for 3-4 minutes until almonds are toasted and beans are coated with oil.
6. Season with salt and pepper to taste. Remove from heat and serve immediately.

## HEALTH BENEFITS

1. Low in calories: Suitable for weight management and overall health.
2. High in fiber: Promotes digestive health and helps with satiety.
3. Rich in vitamins and minerals: Green beans provide vitamin C, vitamin K, and folate.

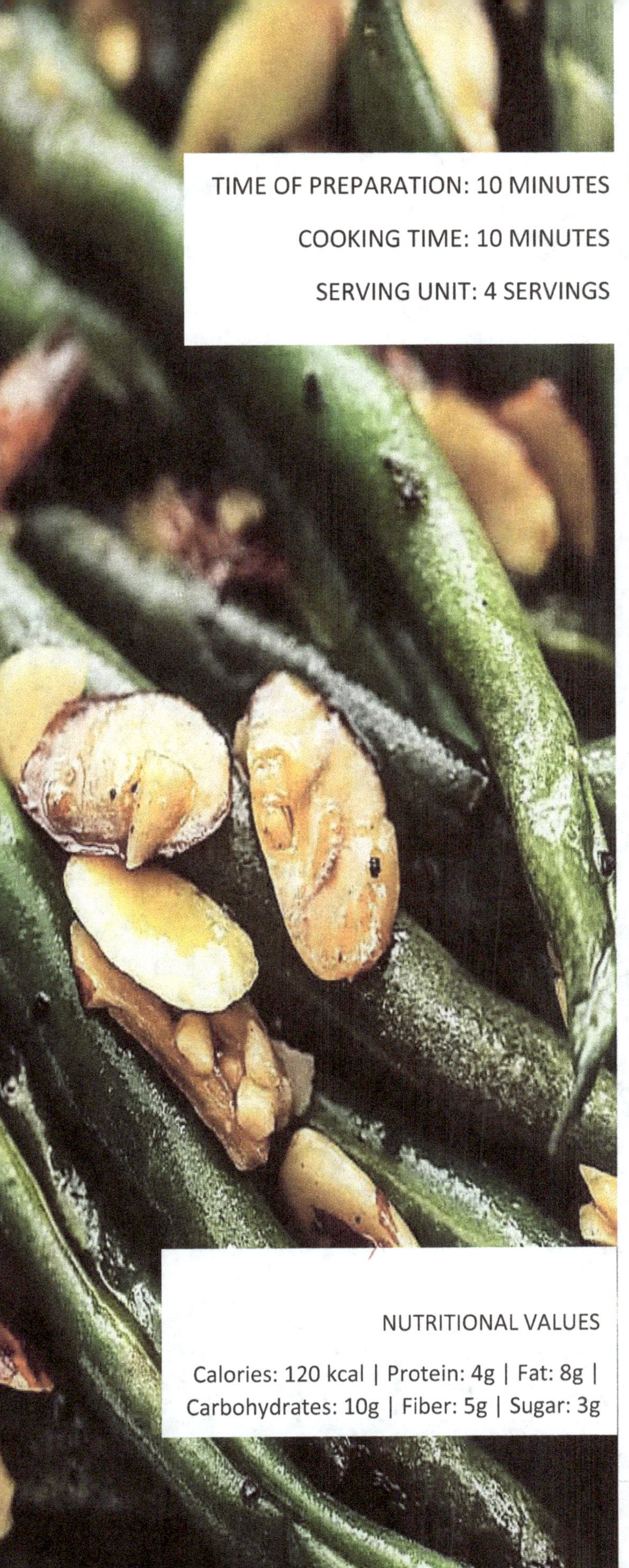

NUTRITIONAL VALUES

Calories: 120 kcal | Protein: 4g | Fat: 8g | Carbohydrates: 10g | Fiber: 5g | Sugar: 3g

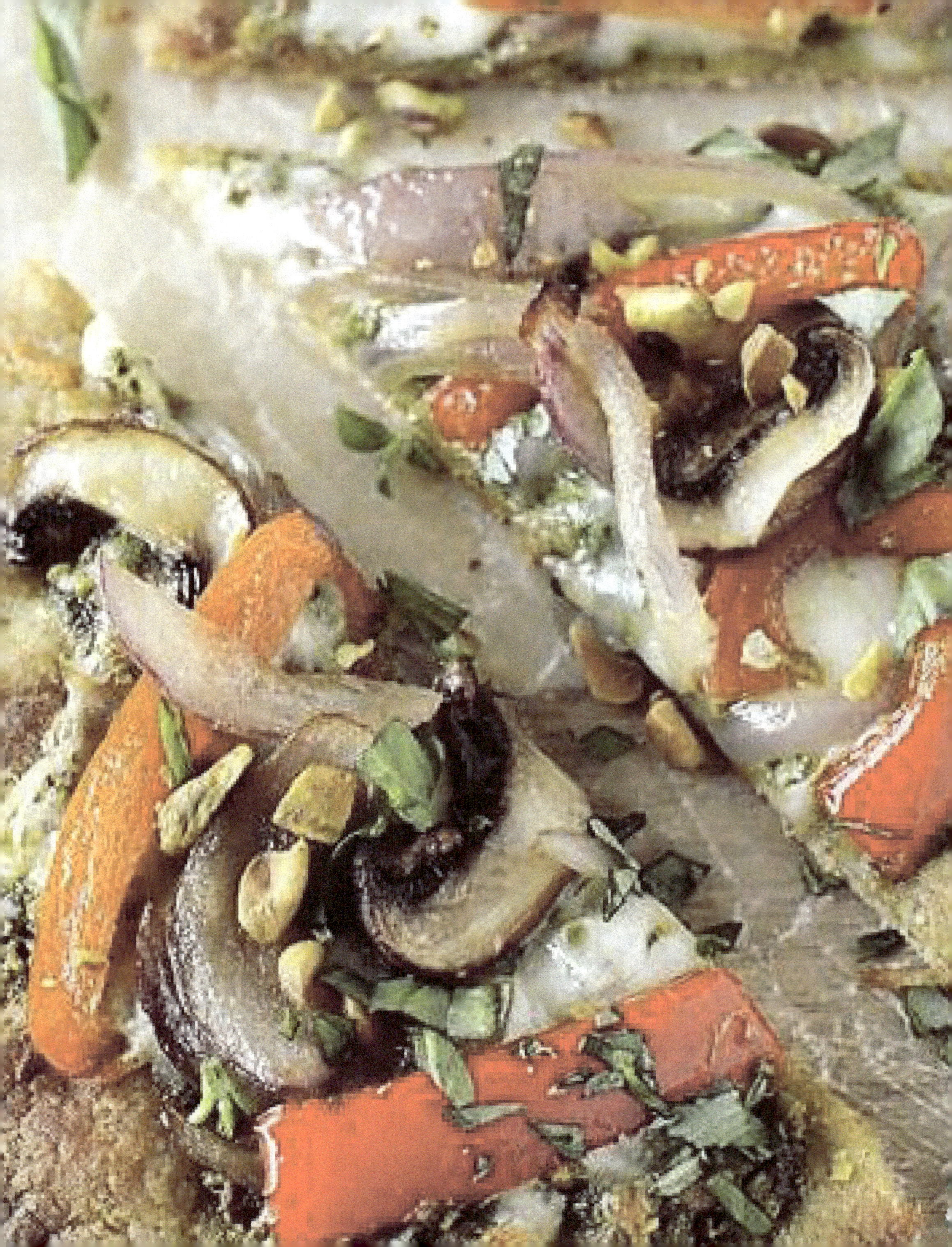

# CONCLUSION

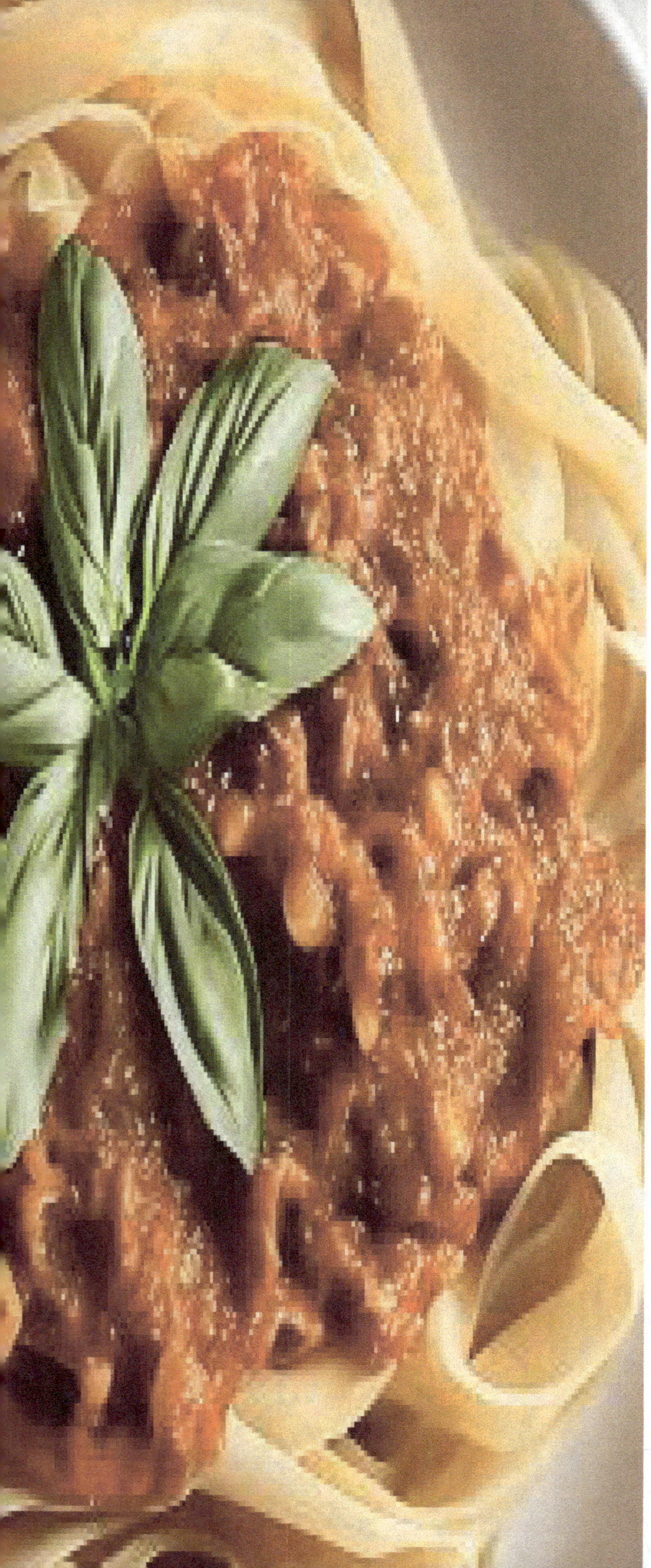



In conclusion, the DASH (Dietary Approaches to Stop Hypertension) diet cookbook offers a wealth of delicious and nutritious recipes designed to promote heart health, lower blood pressure, and support overall well-being. Throughout this cookbook, you've discovered a variety of flavorful dishes that emphasize whole grains, lean proteins, fruits, and vegetables—all essential components of the DASH diet. By incorporating these recipes into your daily meals, you're not only embracing a healthier lifestyle but also enjoying food that is both satisfying and beneficial for your cardiovascular health.

Each recipe in this cookbook has been carefully crafted to meet the dietary guidelines recommended by health professionals, making it easier for you to maintain balanced nutrition without sacrificing taste. Whether you're looking to manage hypertension, improve your heart health, or simply adopt a more wholesome diet, the DASH diet cookbook provides practical solutions and delicious inspirations.

# CELEBRATING YOUR DASH DIET JOURNEY

As you conclude your journey with the DASH diet, take a moment to celebrate your achievements and commitment to health. Whether you've embraced new recipes, made dietary adjustments, or experienced positive changes in your well-being, every step counts towards better health. Celebrate the small victories—trying new ingredients, mastering cooking techniques, or discovering flavors that nourish both body and soul.

Your journey with the DASH diet is not just about food; it's about creating sustainable habits that support a healthier lifestyle. As you continue on this path, remember to listen to your body, enjoy the process of preparing and savoring nutritious meals, and appreciate the benefits of making informed choices for your health.

# STAYING MOTIVATED AND INSPIRED FOR DASH DIET

- **SET REALISTIC GOALS:** Break down your goals into achievable steps. Celebrate each milestone, whether it's trying a new recipe or incorporating more vegetables into your meals.
- **VARIETY IS KEY:** Explore different recipes and flavors to keep your meals interesting and enjoyable. Experiment with seasonal produce and diverse cooking techniques to add excitement to your diet.
- **STAY INFORMED:** Stay updated with the latest nutrition research and guidelines. Understanding the health benefits of the foods you eat can reinforce your commitment to the DASH diet.
- **MEAL PLANNING:** Plan your meals ahead of time to ensure you have nutritious options readily available. This can help prevent impulse eating and make healthy choices more accessible.
- **FIND SUPPORT:** Join online communities, support groups, or involve family and friends in your journey. Sharing experiences and tips can provide encouragement and motivation.
- **MINDFUL EATING:** Practice mindful eating by paying attention to hunger and fullness cues. Enjoy each bite, savoring the flavors and textures of your food.
- **CELEBRATE SUCCESSES:** Acknowledge your progress and successes along the way. Whether it's improved energy levels, better blood pressure readings, or simply feeling more vibrant, celebrate these achievements.

*By staying motivated and inspired, you can continue to embrace the principles of the DASH diet and enjoy the lifelong benefits of a balanced and healthful eating pattern. Remember, every positive choice you make contributes to your overall well-being and vitality.*

# TIPS FOR LONG-TERM SUCCESS ON THE DASH DIET

1. **GRADUAL TRANSITION:** Start by making small changes to your diet and lifestyle. Gradually incorporate more fruits, vegetables, whole grains, and lean proteins into your meals.

2. **PORTION CONTROL:** Pay attention to portion sizes to avoid overeating, especially with foods high in calories, sodium, or unhealthy fats.

3. **STAY HYDRATED:** Drink plenty of water throughout the day. Water helps regulate body temperature, aids digestion, and supports overall health.

4. **REDUCE SODIUM INTAKE:** Limit processed foods and choose low-sodium options whenever possible. Use herbs, spices, and citrus juices to flavor foods instead of salt.

5. **REGULAR PHYSICAL ACTIVITY:** Incorporate regular exercise into your routine. Aim for at least 150 minutes of moderate-intensity aerobic activity or 75 minutes of vigorous activity each week, as recommended by health guidelines.

6. **MINDFUL EATING:** Practice mindful eating by focusing on the present moment and paying attention to hunger and fullness cues. Avoid distractions while eating, such as watching TV or using electronic devices.

7. **PLAN AND PREPARE MEALS:** Plan your meals ahead of time and prepare healthy snacks to avoid making impulsive food choices. This can help you stay on track with your dietary goals.

8. **SEEK SUPPORT:** Surround yourself with supportive friends, family members, or a healthcare professional who can encourage and motivate you on your journey.

9. **MONITOR PROGRESS:** Track your progress by keeping a food diary or using a nutrition app to monitor your daily intake and physical activity. Celebrate your successes and learn from challenges.

10. **LIFELONG COMMITMENT:** Understand that the DASH diet is not a temporary fix but a lifelong commitment to health. Embrace the principles of balanced nutrition, moderation, and regular physical activity for sustained well-being.

# EMBRACING A HEALTHIER FUTURE WITH THE DASH DIET

***Here are key steps to embrace a healthier future with the DASH diet***

1. **NUTRIENT-RICH FOODS:** Focus on nutrient-dense foods that provide essential vitamins, minerals, and antioxidants to support overall health and vitality.

2. **BALANCED NUTRITION:** Maintain a balanced diet by incorporating a variety of foods from different food groups to ensure you're getting a wide range of nutrients.

3. **HEART HEALTH:** Prioritize heart health by choosing foods that help lower blood pressure and reduce the risk of cardiovascular diseases, such as hypertension.

4. **LIFESTYLE CHANGES:** Adopt healthy lifestyle habits, including regular physical activity, adequate hydration, stress management, and sufficient sleep.

5. **EDUCATIONAL RESOURCES:** Stay informed about nutrition guidelines, healthy cooking methods, and portion control to make informed choices for your diet.

6. **COMMUNITY SUPPORT:** Seek support from friends, family, or online communities to stay motivated, share experiences, and learn new recipes and tips.

***By embracing the DASH diet as a sustainable way of eating, you're paving the way for a healthier future filled with energy, vitality, and well-being. Each positive choice you make contributes to a lifestyle that supports longevity and quality of life.***

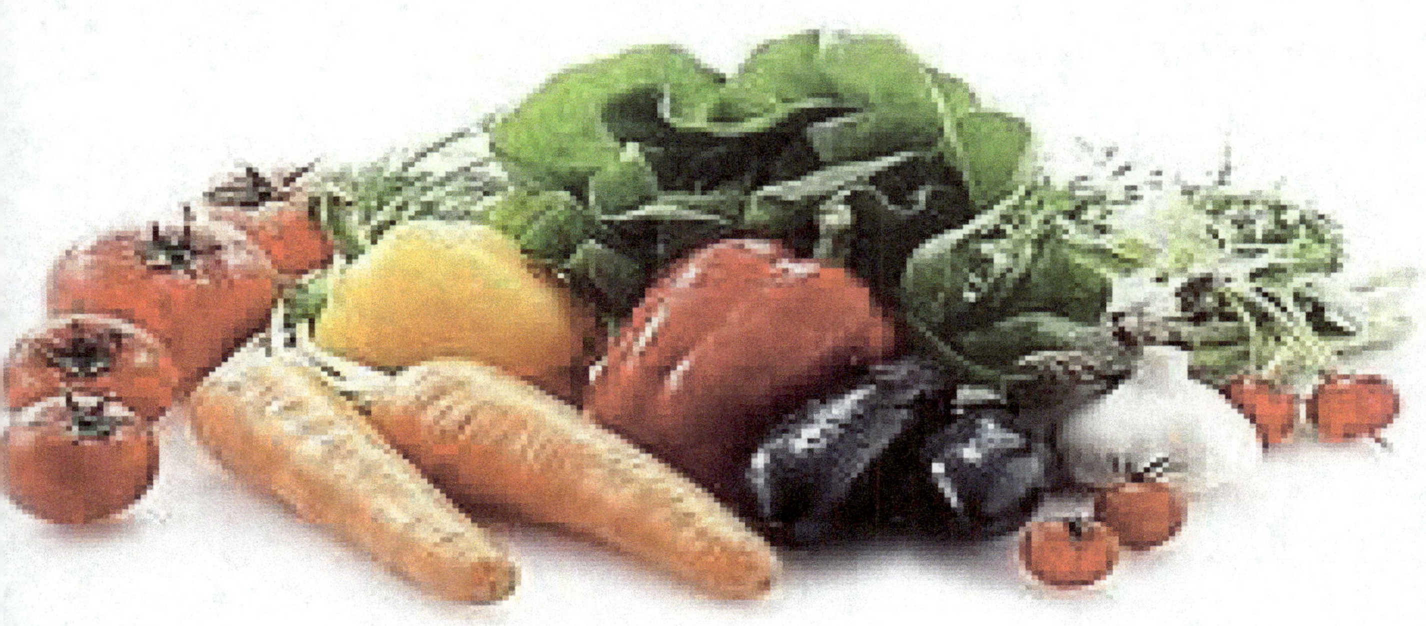

# 14-DAY MEAL PLANNING

## DAY 1

Breakfast: Berry Overnight Oats

Lunch: Greek Salad Skewers

Dinner: Grilled Salmon with Lemon-Dill Sauce

Snack: Fruit and Nut Energy Bites

## DAY 2

Breakfast: Spinach and Feta Omelet

Lunch: Lentil and Vegetable Soup

Dinner: Quinoa-Stuffed Bell Peppers

Snack: Mixed Green Beans with Almonds

## DAY 3

Breakfast: Banana Nut Pancakes

Lunch: Mediterranean Quinoa Salad

Dinner: Chicken and Vegetable Stir-Fry

Snack: Greek Yogurt Parfait with Fresh Fruits

## DAY 4

Breakfast: Greek Yogurt Parfait with Fresh Fruits

Lunch: Sweet Potato and Black Bean Chili

Dinner: Baked Cod with Herb Crust

Snack: Hummus and Veggie Platter

## DAY 5

Breakfast: Quinoa Breakfast Bowl

| |
|---|
| Lunch: Kale and Apple Salad with Walnuts |
| Dinner: Lentil and Mushroom Shepherd's Pie |
| Snack: Berry Blast Smoothie |
| |

## DAY 6

| |
|---|
| Breakfast: Golden Turmeric Latte |
| Lunch: Tomato Basil Soup |
| Dinner: Grilled Chicken Caesar Salad |
| Snack: Cucumber Mint Water |
| |

## DAY 7

| |
|---|
| Breakfast: Berry Blast Smoothie |
| Lunch: Minestrone Soup |
| Dinner: Quinoa-Stuffed Bell Peppers |
| Snack: Fruit and Nut Energy Bites |
| |

## DAY 8

| |
|---|
| Breakfast: Avocado Toast with Tomato and Basil |
| Lunch: Spinach, Strawberry, and Almond Salad |
| Dinner: Hearty Chicken and Barley Stew |
| Snack: Garlic and Herb Roasted Vegetables |

## DAY 9

| |
|---|
| Breakfast: Mixed Green Beans with Almonds |
| Lunch: Chickpea and Cucumber Salad |
| Dinner: Steamed Asparagus with Lemon Zest |
| Snack: Brown Rice Pilaf |

## DAY 10

Breakfast: Berry Overnight Oats

Lunch: Hummus and Veggie Platter

Dinner: Lentil and Vegetable Soup

Snack: Fruit and Nut Energy Bites

## DAY 11

Breakfast: Quinoa Breakfast Bowl

Lunch: Greek Salad Skewers

Dinner: Chicken and Vegetable Stir-Fry

Snack: Cucumber Mint Water

## DAY 12

Breakfast: Greek Yogurt Parfait with Fresh Fruits

Lunch: Mediterranean Quinoa Salad

Dinner: Grilled Salmon with Lemon-Dill Sauce

Snack: Mixed Green Beans with Almonds

## DAY 13

Breakfast: Banana Nut Pancakes

Lunch: Kale and Apple Salad with Walnuts

Dinner: Lentil and Mushroom Shepherd's Pie

Snack: Greek Yogurt Parfait with Fresh Fruits

## DAY 14

| |
|---|
| Breakfast: Golden Turmeric Latte |
| Lunch: Tomato Basil Soup |
| Dinner: Quinoa-Stuffed Bell Peppers |
| Snack: Hummus and Veggie Platter |

*This 14-day meal plan incorporates a variety of delicious and nutritious recipes aligned with the DASH diet principles. Each day includes balanced meals and snacks rich in fruits, vegetables, lean proteins, whole grains, and heart-healthy fats. Adjust portion sizes and ingredients based on individual dietary needs and preferences.*

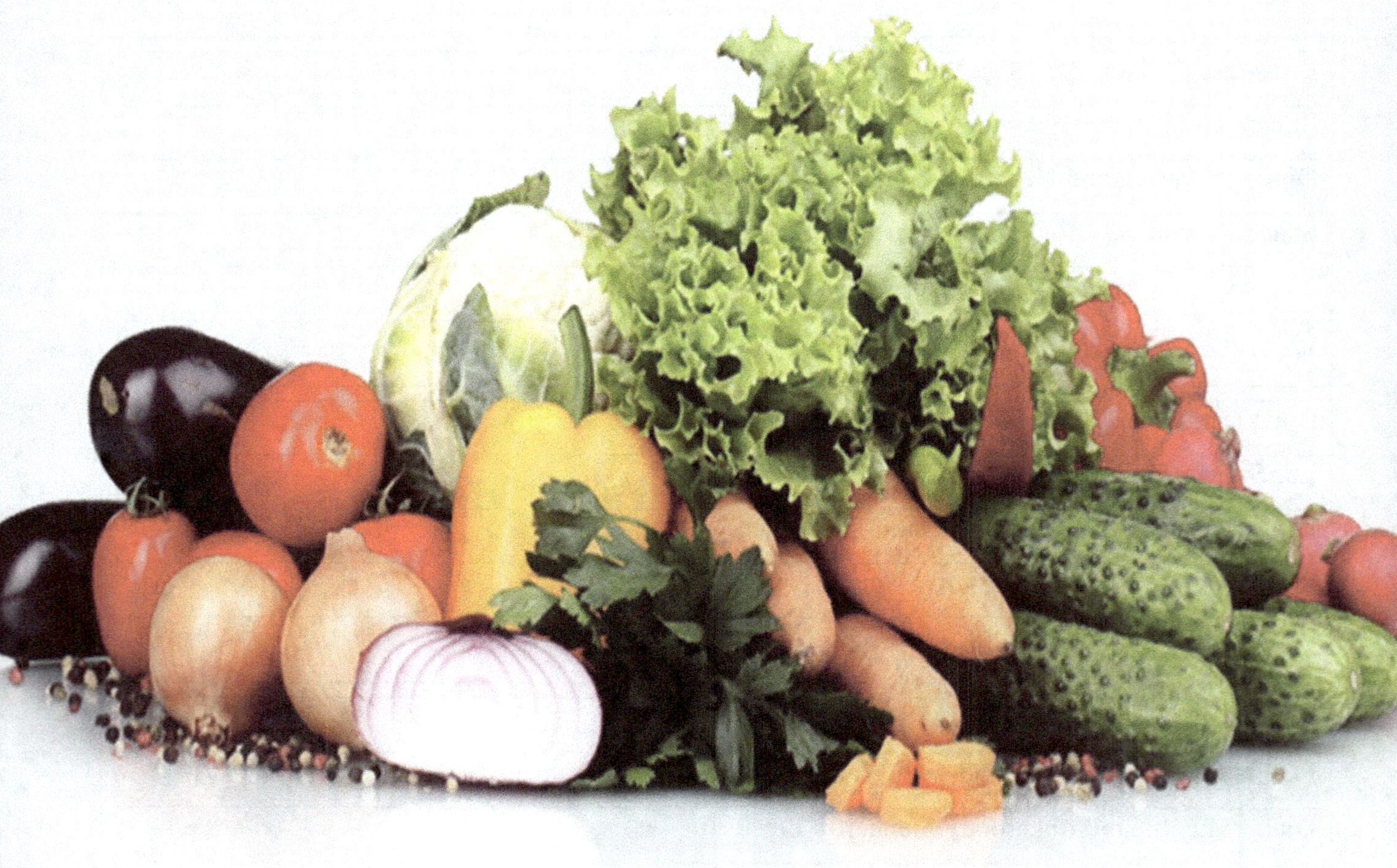

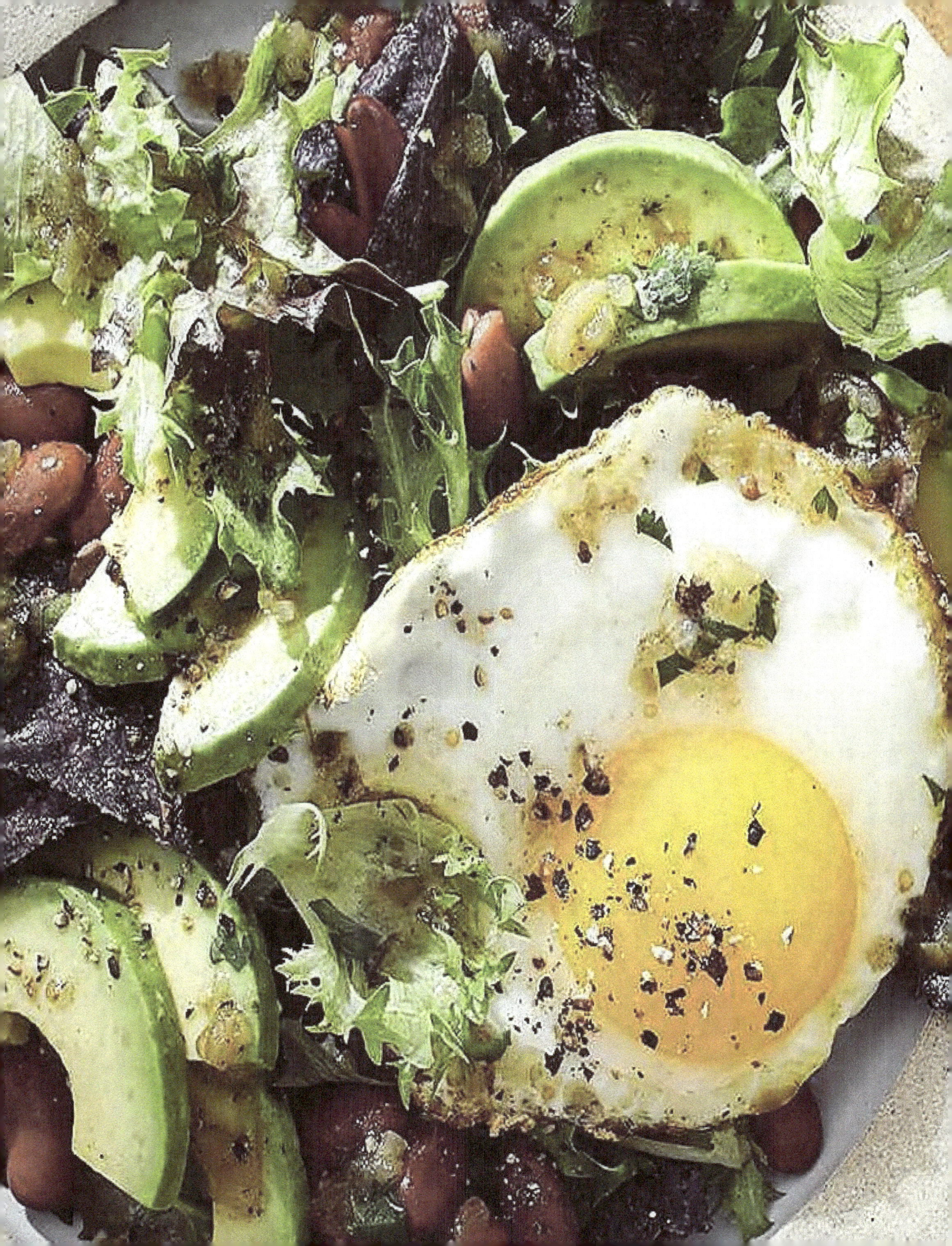

# INDEX

## A

Avocado Toast with Tomato and Basil

## B

Banana Nut Pancakes

Berry Blast Smoothie

Berry Overnight Oats

Brown Rice Pilaf

## C

Chickpea and Cucumber Salad

Chicken and Vegetable Stir-Fry

Cucumber Mint Water

## G

Garlic and Herb Roasted Vegetables

Golden Turmeric Latte

Greek Salad Skewers

Greek Yogurt Parfait with Fresh Fruits

Grilled Chicken Caesar Salad

Grilled Salmon with Lemon-Dill Sauce

## H

Hearty Chicken and Barley Stew

Hummus and Veggie Platter

## K

Kale and Apple Salad with Walnuts

## L

Lentil and Mushroom Shepherd's Pie

Lentil and Vegetable Soup

## M

Mediterranean Quinoa Salad

Minestrone Soup

Mixed Green Beans with Almonds

## Q

Quinoa Breakfast Bowl

Quinoa-Stuffed Bell Peppers

## S

Spinach and Feta Omelet

Spinach, Strawberry, and Almond Salad

Steamed Asparagus with Lemon Zest

Sweet Potato and Black Bean Chili

T

Tomato Basil Soup